The Working Woman's Body Book

The Working Woman's Body Book

Lilian Rowen

with

Barbara Winkler

Illustrated by Ron Jones

Rawson Associates Publishers, Inc.
New York

Library of Congress Cataloging in Publication Data

Rowen, Lilian.
The working woman's body book.

Includes index.
1. Exercise for women. I. Winkler, Barbara,
joint author. II. Title.
GV482.R68 1978   613.7′045   77–17644
ISBN 0–89256–055–X
ISBN 0–89256–059–2 pbk.

Published simultaneously in Canada by McClelland
and Stewart, Ltd.
Manufactured in the United States of America
by
American Book–Stratford Press, Inc.
Saddle Brook, New Jersey

Designed by Gene Siegel
First Edition

To my husband Mel,
and of course,
to working women everywhere

Foreword

There is not enough exercise in our mechanized society and tensions in our lives are greater than ever.

These facts have contributed to a number of diseases such as myocardial infarctions, duodenal ulcers, diabetes, overweight, neurosis, and back and neck ache. It has therefore become imperative to develop the habits of exercise and relaxation as a means to keep us healthy.

Miss Rowen's book will be a valuable contribution to these preventive measures. Exercise to keep the muscles of the body in good shape, to relax, and to add a minimum of cardiovascular workout are described in her book.

Descriptions of exercises are clear, easy to follow, and are aided by excellent illustrations. The material is well organized.

It is my pleasure to recommend this book to all women who realize that early exercise and relaxation are as necessary as a healthy diet and sufficient vitamins. It is understood that a visit to their physician should precede the start of any unaccustomed physical activity.

Hans Kraus, M.D.

Medical consultant to the President's
Council on Physical Fitness and Sports

Contents

The Working Woman's Body Book

1

My Program— How It Began and How It Works

Of course, you should exercise regularly. You know that. But all of us who work also know how hard it is to find time for an exercise routine in our busy lives. I've long been aware of this because the clients at my exercise studio in New York are primarily working women. Most regret that their schedules won't permit them to manage more than one or two sessions a week at the studio. Inevitably, after they've become hooked on how much good exercise is doing for them, a familiar query is put to me: "Why doesn't someone come up with an exercise program I can follow *wherever* I am, and that I can change to fit my needs—something that fits *my* life, *my* time?"

I didn't really take this query to heart until the day I found myself browsing through the Health and Beauty section of a bookstore while waiting for my husband. As I looked I found this: exercise books based on dance and yoga; exercises from famous people, famous spas, and military organizations; specialized programs to lengthen your life, improve sex, ease aches and pains; not to mention weight lifting, partner, and water routines. Not *one* of the books spoke to the special needs of the working woman.

That experience started me thinking. And remembering. Back in the 1950s I found it difficult to fit exercise into my own life. I was working at an office job (because the demand for exercise instructors was only beginning to grow), looking for an apartment, taking classes, and dating a great deal.

Sitting at my desk all day was absolute torture—I was itching to move, to bend, to swing—but it seemed that my lifestyle had no room in it for a regular exercise workout. To compensate, I would do desk exercises like the Shoulder Shrug (Chapter 12—Exercises to Do in Places You Never Thought of), but stopped when I overheard a co-worker saying to someone else, "I wonder what's wrong with Lilian? She's always shaking."

I then started to do coffee break exercises in the ladies room (usually the Bouncing Body, Chorus Line Kick and/or Knee Kicker—all in Chapter 6, Stamina Build-Ups), and at lunch I'd do some fast walking. Whenever possible, I'd exercise at home, but wasn't able to as often as I would have liked. Luckily, I soon got a job teaching exercise classes.

So, looking back on my own experience, I was struck by the real need for a program that would meet a working woman's special requirements. The prerequisites were: personalization, flexibility, ease, and a short amount of time. And my clients added another—fun. Most programs, they said, get so boring that they're hard to stick with. Armed with my knowledge of my students' needs and my long experience supervising such programs in the studio, I set to work to design a *personalized,* portable, speedy program. The result is this book.

What My Program Is

The Working Woman's Body Program is based on personalized exercise workouts that you plan and design yourself. You do the exercises you need for your body and state of mind. And you do them eclectically. Technique is not glorified because I've found that it is the effort, not the form, that makes for improvement. And, if you skip a day here and there, then exercise for 13 minutes the next day, and 26 minutes the day after, the same principle still applies. As long as there is *effort,* there will be results. As for fun, the exercises are designed in such a way that they can be alternated and switched around at will, so they *never* get boring. Because the program includes different types of exercises, such as yoga stretches and jazz warm-ups, you get to try a wide variety of movements, which makes it more interesting.

How My Program Works

Most exercise routines have a specific set of exercises that you do over and over every day. Not this one. You choose which exercises you want from a pool of over 100 and change them around whenever you feel like it. Although you should aim for a weekly exercise quota of roughly 90 minutes, how you slot this time is entirely up to you. On days when you're short of time, you can take as little as 13 minutes to work out; on days when you're not as busy, you can add new exercises or increase the amount of time you do your favorites. And—this may come as a shocker—you don't have to exercise daily. To start an exercise program with the idea that you must do it faithfully every day is psychologically discouraging. Skip a day or two if your schedule demands it or your head can't take it. As long as you don't play hooky for more than two days, you're still okay and won't lose muscle elasticity.

In order to find out what your trouble spots are and which exercises will help correct them, take the Working Woman's Body Quiz in Chapter 3. Then, look over all the exercises, and start designing your routine. The exercises are organized by chapter into the following categories:

The Preparation

· Warm-Ups (Chapter 4)—to prepare your muscles for exercising

The Workout

· Figure Improvers/Strengtheners (Chapter 5)—to spot-reduce problem areas by firming and strengthening the muscles
· Stamina Build-Ups (Chapter 6)—to increase endurance by strengthening the heart and improving lung function
· Flexibility Exercises (Chapter 7)—to increase muscle elasticity and stretch ligaments for a more supple body and more graceful movements

· Tension Releasers (Chapter 8)—to relax muscles and mind so you can cope with the stress of a working lifestyle
· Posture/Balance Fixers (Chapter 9)—to learn body alignment so you can hold yourself properly and confidently

The Wind-Up

· Cool-Offs (Chapter 10)—to return muscles to their normal, unexcited state

You prepare for your individual program with 3 minutes of Warm-Ups and wind up with 2 minutes of Cool-Offs for health reasons, but that is the only routine you have to follow. The middle part of the program—the workout—is entirely up to you. This is where you focus on your particular body problems and choose the exercises to correct them. How you divide the time between the various categories depends on your individual needs. However, if you are including the Tension Releasers in your workout, do them *immediately* after the Warm-Ups.

When designing your workout, consider your particular needs at that time. For instance, if you've been locked in at your desk all day, or sitting in a long series of meetings, chuck your usual Figure Improvers/Strengtheners and concentrate on more Warm-Ups For People Who Sit All Day or Stamina Build-Ups. Or, if bikini time is coming up, add to your waist and stomach exercises and limit your Stamina Build-Ups. Remember, flexibility is a keynote of the program, but it is up to you to take advantage of it.

To understand how my system works, here is one client's routine: she's an executive secretary, healthy, about the right weight, but has a bulge on her upper thighs and her waist is not as small as she would like it to be. She comes home from a hard day at the office where she's been at her desk typing and taking notes at meetings, is tired and tense and has a dinner date at 8:00, so time is limited. Her exercise plan: 1 minute for the Basic Body Relaxer Warm-Up and 2 minutes of Jazzaerobic Warm-Ups (good for people who sit all day), 2 minutes of Tension Releasers to unwind, 6 minutes of waist and thigh improvers, and 2 minutes of Cool-Off movements. Result: in 13 minutes she's worked on her trouble spots, loosened up, and relaxed. The following day when she's not as tense, and has more time, she can eliminate the Tension Releasers and substitute 2 minutes of Posture Fixers, add 3 minutes of Flexibility Exercises and do 4 more minutes of Figure Improvers/Strengtheners for a more thorough, 20-minute workout.

For other ideas on how to personalize the program to suit your needs, look at the Situation Chart, in Chapter 13. It outlines programs for specific working-woman problems—those once-every-so-often situations that turn up like Hard Day at the Office, Kinked Up and Stiff, Hard Day Ahead. Keep in mind, however, that the routines on that chart are not outlines for daily personal workouts. They are for special occasions.

Because your lifestyle is bound to change from time to time, there is also a chapter on Specialty Exercises, which include Pre-Ski and Pre-Tennis routines, a Jogging Curriculum, a Post-Natal Shape-Up and Menstrual Soothers. These are all easy mini-programs that can be done by themselves, or, in the case of the sport exercises, in addition to your regular regimen. Then, to make even better use of your time, there's a chapter on exercises to do in places you never thought of. Examine it for ideas on exercising at the beach, in the tub, at your desk, and other surprising spots.

One more point. Although the exercises here are not harmful in any way, you never should start an exercise program without first checking with your physician.

How to Make This Program Work Best for You

Here are some tips that will help you get the most out of my program; study it before you begin:

1. For freedom of movement, wear as few clothes as possible. A leotard or T-shirt and bikini panties are both good ideas. The important thing is to have nothing restricting around your waist and to take off your bra unless you are very large-breasted and need the support.

2. Exercise to music. Most anything is fine because of the encouraging psychological effect, but disco, rock, or jazz all have an easily identifiable beat that will help you keep a steady

rhythm. If you are doing the Tension Release program, switch to something slow and easy like Chopin or Mozart.

3. As you exercise, be sure you are breathing properly. You should exhale at the difficult or strenuous part of *each* exercise and the exhalation should be done through your mouth. Breathlessness only occurs when you hold too much air in and your lungs get so filled up that you become uncomfortable. To alleviate this, concentrate on exhaling until nothing is left in your lungs; don't worry about the inhaling because you will do it automatically.

4. Keep in mind that it is the *effort* that counts, not the technique. With each exercise, go into your furthest stretch, your highest kick, your deepest bend. As long as you are doing the best you can, the fact that you don't look perfect has very little meaning.

5. Each time you do an exercise and return to starting position between counts, go limp and relax all over; then begin again and use your muscles to the utmost. It is this relax-then-act syndrome that strengthens, shapes, and firms.

6. The amount of time given for each exercise is a minimum count. Start off with this amount and increase gradually as your body becomes more supple. Do not, however, increase to more than double the amount given.

7. Where time spans are given, the amounts are approximate. Much depends on your individual speed and body weight, so if you fall a bit short or need a little more time, don't worry.

8. Never exercise right after a meal—wait at least an hour or so for your food to settle. If you are dieting, it's a good idea to exercise immediately before a meal. Contrary to what you may have heard about exercise increasing your appetite, you will find that it actually curbs it. Experiment—you'll see!

9. Don't be concerned about not exercising at the same time each day. The only validity to the "same-time-same-place" theory is that it does build a habit.

10. Don't forget to re-evaluate your needs regularly and change your program to fit them.

11. Once you have shaped up to your pleasure, work out an all-around program that includes Stamina and Flexibility Exercises and Tension Releasers to maintain your fitness.

12. If you haven't been exercising at all and find it painful,

start off with only a few minutes every day. Do this for about 2 weeks, then work out a longer program and feel free to skip a day every so often. You might work up to the "I've Never Done Exercises Before" routine on the Situation Chart.

2

The Philosophy
Behind My Program

Now that you're familiar with the program, you're bound to have some questions. Why does it work? What is the theory behind it? How is it possible to get benefits if you exercise only one and a half hours a week? And why should you do it over some other program?

For starters, let's take the last question. The Working Woman's Body Program is the best for you not only because of its personalization and flexibility, but because it's geared to a total body approach. Fitness as well as shaping up is the aim. To achieve this dual goal, four things must be accomplished.

1. *Strengthening muscles,* which in turn firms and tones them
2. *Building up stamina* to achieve better performance of your cardio-pulmonary system
3. *Increasing flexibility* for a more supple body and more co-ordinated movements
4. *Learning muscle relaxation* and eliminating tension

The Working Woman's Body Program fulfills all these goals. Besides working toward a specific end, such as increasing endurance, the exercises have been designed to interact and build

10

on each other. And the addition of both a Posture and a Tension Release program means that a truly better working body, a body in absolute prime condition, will be the result.

But, you may ask, I jog five times a week, so why do this? Or perhaps you do yoga or isometrics? These are fine in combination with the program, but alone are not enough because they neglect certain important areas. Although you may be using specific muscles in these other exercises, that does not necessarily mean that those muscles are being strengthened. In fact, many times the using is really abusing. To evaluate how other programs and sports affect your body, look over the following breakdown:

Aerobics: Terrific for cardio-pulmonary efficiency; strengthens certain areas depending on which exercises you do; no effect on flexibility or muscle relaxation; does release mental tension

Isometrics: Contracts and eventually cramps muscles; works for strength (firming) only; no flexibility or muscle relaxation; does not improve the working of your cardio-pulmonary system; no effect on tension release

Yoga: Good for flexibility, toning, and muscle relaxation; leaves out cardio-pulmonary improvement entirely; relieves tension

Weight lifting: Creates strength in the muscles but does not stretch and relax them at all; no effect on the cardio-pulmonary system or flexibility; can relieve tension to some degree

Rope skipping: Very hard on feet and knees, especially when done in improper shoes or bare feet; good for cardio-pulmonary efficiency; does not increase flexibility; no strengthening except in legs; does not relax muscles; does release tension

Dance: Most dance programs concentrate on stretches and neglect strengthening of the stomach and back; good for flexibility and cardio-pulmonary efficiency; does not teach muscle relaxation; releases mental tension somewhat

Jogging: Good for your cardio-pulmonary system, but has no effect on flexibility or muscle relaxation; uses back and stomach muscles, but does not strengthen them and sometimes can even hurt them; the action involved does help relieve tension

Tennis: Hard on back and elbows and shoulders; does increase cardio-pulmonary efficiency; strengthens legs and one arm;

minimum effect on flexibility; can create tension instead of releasing it; no effect on muscle relaxation

Skiing: Very strenuous sport that's good for building up cardio-pulmonary efficiency and strengthening legs; not good for flexibility or muscle relaxation; uses back and stomach muscles, but does not strengthen them; can relieve tension

Golf: No flexibility, strengthening, or muscle relaxing effects; some cardio-pulmonary improvement if you walk; very often it tends to create tension

Bicycling: Good for strengthening legs and increasing cardio-pulmonary efficiency; not good for flexibility, stomach or back strengthening, or muscle relaxation; good tension releaser

Skating: Good for strengthening legs and some benefit to back and stomach muscles; no effect on muscle relaxation or flexibility; does improve cardio-pulmonary performance; releases tension

Swimming: A total body sport; done correctly it is the most valid sport exercise because it stretches, strengthens, improves cardio-pulmonary efficiency, increases flexibility, relaxes muscles, and releases tension. The only drawback is that you need access to a pool. For most of us, the time needed to get to a pool and in and out of a bathing suit is too long

Housework: Does involve some stretching and bending, but these are spasmodic movements and can be harmful to weak backs; does not improve flexibility or cardio-pulmonary performance; has no effect on muscle relaxation; very often creates tension.

You can carry out the Working Woman's Body Program in your home, or even in your office if you have the privacy—you don't have to do it in a pool, on a court, or outside on the street. You don't need any special equipment. And it works on your entire body.

As for the factors of personalization and flexibility, they stem from my belief that exercise should be as individual as medication. Many programs are much too general. In Austria, where I studied, the training was geared to the individual. In my classes I concentrate on what each student wants and needs, whether it be exercises to trim down "office spread" or posture and flexibility improvement.

Each woman works at her own pace and I always give supplementary routines to do at home. For example, I have a client who is an illustrator and works at home. She is bent over drawings for long periods of time, so to unkink her muscles, I devised this 13-minute "refresher" for her: 1 minute of the Basic Body Relaxer, 2 minutes of either the Jogger or the Jazzaerobics Warm-Ups, 3 minutes of lying down Figure Improvers/Strengtheners (The Cycler, The Crossover, The Triple Threat), 3 minutes of the Stamina Build-Ups of her choice, 2 minutes of Flexibility Exercises (the Pectoral Stretch, Shoulder Pull, Rocking Horse, Zipper Pull), and a 2-minute wind-up with the Rag Doll Series of Cool-Offs. This routine reverses the bent-over, sitting down position she's been in, gets her circulation going, stretches her leg muscles, and just generally unkinks her body.

Another client has a very different problem. She's a real estate agent and is constantly running around showing apartments. All this activity takes its toll on her back and legs and she often finds herself aching—not to mention tense and wound up —at the end of the day. She comes to my studio twice a week for an overall workout, plays tennis whenever she can, and follows this mini-program that I planned for her at home: she starts off with the 5-minute Tension Release program to relax her muscles and her mind, then goes into her personal workout, which includes 3 minutes of Warm-Ups For People Who Are on Their Feet All Day, 2 minutes of Figure Improvers (the Knee Bounce, the Triple Threat, the Crossover), 1½ minutes of Flexibility Exercises (Heel Stretch, Sole Clapper, Back Stretcher) and finishes off with the Sit-Down Coolers. This program releases tension, relaxes her leg and back muscles, and works on improving back and hamstring flexibility. She also does the Ankle Flexer whenever possible during the course of her working day.

The exercise programs in this book offer the same kinds of personalization that I've worked out for these two women—the only difference is that *you* do the planning. You pick what you need and disregard the rest. The Body Quiz (Chapter 3) shows you how to do the planning for your specific needs.

Another point that probably needs explaining is the time element. It is based on two very sound principles: 1) that exercise works cumulatively when done regularly, and 2) that most of you who work have enough exercise built into your lifestyles so that you don't need to spend an extraordinary amount of time on a daily program.

Once you exercise on a regular basis, each exercise builds on what has been done before. Because muscles are constantly being stretched and strengthened, they don't have a chance to atrophy. By exercising with some regularity, you create a reservoir of fitness that you constantly add to. However, if you work out only once a week, there's no reservoir to build on because your muscles lose tone. So, why are you allowed to skip an occasional day? A day or two off does not ruin the cumulative effect as long as you *usually* work out regularly and never skip more than two days in a row.

Recent research shows that only athletes need large doses of supplementary exercises to keep in top competitive shape. Most normal, healthy people get enough exercise in day-to-day living to maintain their present level of fitness. And since you're not an athlete, and only want a better body, not a competitive one, a small amount of carefully chosen extra exercise is all you really need to keep in shape. Roughly thirteen minutes a day will give you this because it is enough time for your muscles to warm up, realize the effects of exercising, and cool off. A shorter workout won't push your muscles to the limit; a longer one is terrific, but not necessary to maintain the cumulative effect.

A word on the Tension Release chapter. This is included because tension is so much a part of a working woman's life. When you can't scream at your boss, when you must be tactful, when co-workers are driving you crazy, there is a physiological effect along with a psychological one. Your muscles cramp up and eventually go into spasms. The cramped muscles can be in your back, your neck, your stomach; it depends on where your personal sore spot is. You may not feel the effects immediately, but you will as the tension accumulates. For this reason, I recommend *always* starting off your routine with the Basic Body Relaxer. Although it is technically a tension-releasing exercise, it is a warm-up to warming up, and gives your muscles a chance to stretch and relax. If you pull at the muscles with immediate vigorous exercise, they will tighten up even more. As for the Tension Releasers, I strongly advise that some of them be included in your program at least twice a week.

Last—but definitely not least—I want to say something about

diet. Since a good, healthy, working body depends on what you eat as well as how you exercise, a section on diet is also included in this book. It is not, however, a diet in the usual sense. Like exercising, I believe that eating is a very individual thing and do not advocate any strict day-by-day plan. Instead, this chapter gives down-to-earth, practical eating advice that focuses on a working woman's specific problems, such as the business meal, eating on the run, or brown-bagging it. There are how-to-cope guidelines on those special situations that all we working women share which will help you maintain or lose weight. There is also a mini-crash diet to help you shed a few pounds. Skim through it whether or not you're overweight, because you're sure to pick up a tip or two.

Now it is time to take the Body Quiz. Answer the questions honestly and then plan your routine. You'll find that the program is enjoyable, and even more to the point, that it works.

3

The Working Woman's Body Quiz

Do you know what your body problems are? Surprisingly many of my students didn't when they first attended my classes. What one thought was a flabby tummy was really due to bad posture. And another, who was justifiably proud of her figure and came only to maintain it, used to conk out ten minutes before class ended. A third, who stated that she needed to work on her posture, actually needed to improve her flexibility. Her carriage was fine, but she was so stiff that she moved in a rigid, unattractive way. And so, you too may be mistaking one problem for another, or overlooking certain trouble spots altogether.

To help you identify your particular problems—and figure out how to solve them—we've designed the following Body Quiz. The suggestions given, based on your answers, are to be used as a guideline in planning your program. Most important, however, its purpose is to better acquaint you with your body and the behavior that affects your body, so you can get the most out of this book.

What Basic Shape Are You In?

A) Time yourself for 1 minute and alternate jogging in place and jumping from side to side. If you are huffing and puffing at

16

the end of a minute, you need to build up your stamina and should do at least 30 minutes of aerobic exercises each week. You can choose these from the Warm-Ups and Stamina Build-Ups.

B) Take a piece of string as long as you are tall and attach a small weight (a heavy stone or paperweight will do) to the end of it. Tape the top of the string to the top of a full-length mirror. Stand sideways in front of mirror so that the string bisects your ear. If your posture is correct, the line will run from the middle of ear, to middle of shoulder, to middle of hip joint, to middle of ankle. (See sketch.)

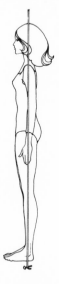

To help correct posture, do the Basic Pelvic Tilt in the various positions. Incorporate 3 to 4 minutes of Back Strengtheners and Flexibility Exercises into your daily workout and use the Posture Reminders whenever possible.

C) Stand up straight, feet together. Bend from hips and try to touch fingertips to floor. If you cannot do this easily, the flexibility of your back and the hamstrings of your legs is a problem, and you should do at least 3 minutes of Flexibility Exercises a day.

D) Lie on back, arms at sides, knees bent, feet on floor. Bring body up into a sitting position. Return to starting position. Do 5 times. If this is difficult, you lack stomach strength, and that could also be the answer to poor posture and/or a protruding stomach. Do at least 3 minutes of stomach exercises from the Figure Improvers chapter every day.

E) Stand up straight, arms at sides. Take one foot off the floor, bend knee, and raise leg until thigh is parallel to floor. Then slowly stand on tiptoe on the other foot and try to hold position for a count of 5.

If you find yourself teeter-tottering, or cannot hold the position for the specified amount of time, you don't have a very good sense of balance. Try to include 2 minutes of Balance Improvers in your daily routine.

How to Uncover Your Trouble Spots

A) The Pinch Test

With your thumb and index finger, grab your body in the following places: tummy, inner upper arms, buttocks, inner thighs.

Wherever you have more than an "inch of pinch," you need firming up. Concentrate on the Figure Improvers for those areas and try to do at least 15 minutes for each of them every week. If you have more than an inch of pinch all over, you are overweight, and need to diet as well as exercise. For tips, read over the diet chapter, but if you must lose a good deal of weight, see your doctor for advice.

B) The Measurement Test

With a tape measure, measure yourself in the following places, and write down the results: wrist, upper arms, bust, waist, thighs, calves, ankles.

Check your results against the following guidelines:

- Upper arm should be 2 times the size of wrist
- Bust should be the same as hips
- Waist should be 10 to 11 inches less than bust
- Thighs should be 6 inches less than waist
- Calves should be 6 to 7 inches less than thighs
- Ankles should be 5 to 6 inches less than calves

Wherever your measurements are more than the standards, there lie your trouble spots. Zero in on them by doing at least 15 minutes of Figure Improvers for each, weekly, until you reach the correct measure.

How to Match Up Your Lifestyle and Your Exercise Needs

A) 1. Are you more of a spectator or a participant in sports?
2. After a day of shopping, do your feet ache?
3. If you run for the bus, or climb a few flights of stairs, do you feel out of breath?
4. Do you get tired after jogging in place for more than 3 minutes?
5. Do you sit at work more than you stand or walk around?

B) 1. Do you have trouble sleeping?
2. Are you often nagged by a headache?

   3. Does your back or neck sometimes ache at the end of the day?
   4. Do you suffer from fatigue?
   5. Do you find yourself getting picky or irritable or blue for no concrete reason?
C) 1. Do you *think* that you get enough exercise?
   2. Is it fairly easy for you to get up in the morning?
   3. If you had a choice between getting a ride to work on a beautiful day, and walking the mile and a half, would you walk?
   4. Are you almost always tired and dragged out after a hard day at work?
   5. During the work week, in the evening, do you prefer to go dancing, bowling, museum hopping, or something else active or would you rather spend the evening at home, seeing a movie, dining out?

A) If you answered "yes" to three or more of the questions in this section, you are a fairly sedentary person and should choose your Warm-Ups accordingly. Do all of your exercises at a comfortable, slightly slow pace and stop the minute you begin to feel tired. Stick with the indicated times for each exercise for the first 2 weeks, then gradually work up to increased amounts and speed. Include several Stamina Build-Ups in your routine.

B) If you answered "yes" to three or more of the questions in this section, you have a tendency to be tense and wound up. Include 3 minutes of Tension Releasers in your daily routine and do the Basic Body Relaxer for 2 minutes instead of 1. About 2 times a week, do the entire 5-minute Tension Release program. Whenever you're in the tub, practice the Deep Breather exercise, and if you sit at a desk most of the day, do the desk exercises to relieve shoulder and neck tension.

C) If you answered "no" to three or more of the questions in this section, you probably need exercise, but don't really want to start an exercise program, even though you know you should. Start off with the Beginner Program explained on the Situation Chart and do it to your favorite music. Or, if you'd rather pick your own exercises, do so, but be sure to include Stamina Build-Ups.

4

Warm-Ups

You've probably heard the term "warm-ups" before, but if you're like most of the women who come to my studio for the first time, you probably have no idea of what it actually means. Warm-ups are exercises that are designed to increase the blood flow to the muscles, so that the muscles literally warm up and become stronger and more flexible. Starting an exercise routine without a few minutes of warm-ups is dangerous because muscles will still be in a cold state and may become cramped.

The Warm-Ups that follow are divided into two categories—for people who are on their feet all day and for those who aren't. Reason: sedentary people need a more active series to warm up because their muscles have been used less. Whichever category you fall into, you must begin your Warm-Ups with the Basic Body Relaxer. This exercise, which takes about a minute, is a general tension releaser that will relax all your muscles and prepare your body for the exercises to follow. This, plus 2 minutes of Warm-Ups, should leave you feeling slightly out of breath. If not, speed up a bit and try to exert more effort. If you get bored repeating the same Warm-Ups every day, alternate them with the Stamina Build-Ups, which have essentially the same result. Just begin with the Basic Body Relaxer, then time yourself for 2 minutes and do the Stamina Build-Ups of your choice.

Basic Body Relaxer

Lie down, flat on back, arms at sides. Close eyes. Breathe deeply, in and out, for a count of 20. Then, let head sink into floor. Let shoulders sink into floor. Right arm. Left arm. Right leg. Left leg. Take a deep breath, in through nose; then exhale through mouth. Move shoulders up and down. Roll head from side to side. Breathe in and out, concentrating on being fully relaxed. Do for 1 minute.

Warm-Ups for People Who Are on Their Feet All Day

The following exercises should be done in the sequence explained here.

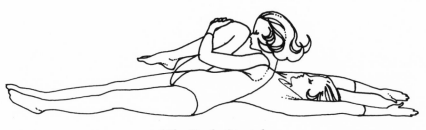

The Body Stretch

Lie flat on back, arms extended above head. Stretch from fingertips to toes, so you feel the pull through your entire body. Then lift head and shoulders up off the floor, bringing arms and back forward. At the same time, bend right knee and bring it up toward your face. Try to touch knee to nose. Return to starting position. Repeat, this time bringing left knee to nose. Do 6 times with each knee.

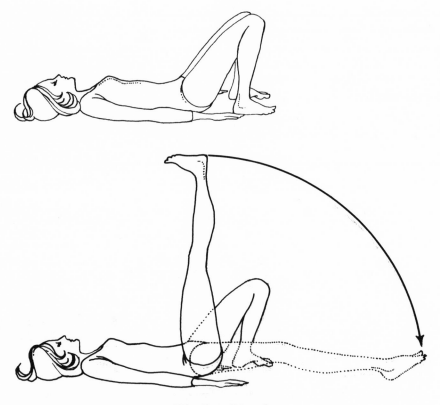

The Leg Stretch

Lie on back with knees bent, arms at sides, feet on floor. Bring right knee up to chest, ankle flexed. Extend leg toward ceiling; relax ankle. Lower leg down to floor. Repeat with left leg. Do 6 times with each leg.

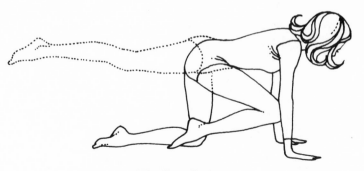

The Leg Swing

Get up onto hands and knees. Swing right leg back and forth fast 6 times, holding leg out straight as it goes back, bending knee up to chest as you bring it forward. Repeat 6 times with left leg.

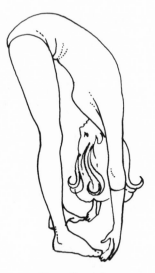

Rest Position

Stand up and let body hang down from hips, arms not quite touching floor. Bounce up and down a few times, breathing slowly and deeply.

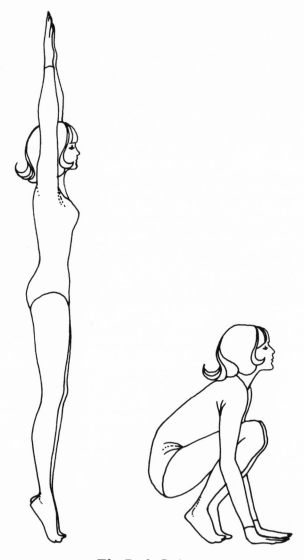

The Body Swing

Stretch upward, bringing arms over head and raising entire body toward ceiling. Swing down quickly into a squatting position, palms touching floor. Start over again with an upward stretch and repeat swings 4 times at a very fast pace. End up in squat position.

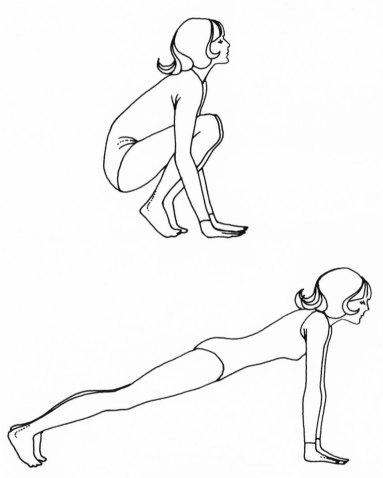

The Body Walk

From the squatting position, walk forward on hands until body is straight. Then walk backward on hands until you reach squatting position again. Repeat 4 times.

Warm-Ups for People Who Sit All Day

Choose either of the following exercises and do for 2 minutes. It's a good idea to use a timer until you become more familiar with your speed.

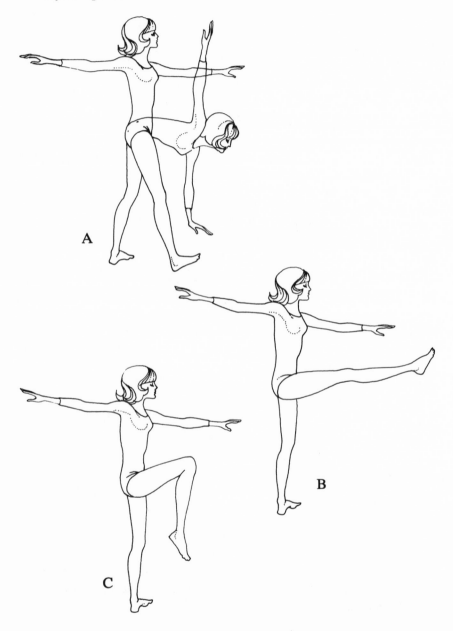

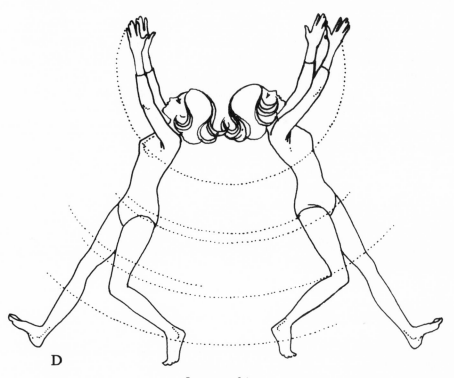

Jazzaerobics

Do the following sequence of steps at a vigorous pace to music. A) Stand up, step forward on right heel, bring foot back; step forward on left heel, bring foot back. Move arms in time with feet as you step, bringing one forward, one back. As you move, lower your body, using 8 counts to get body in position where left hand will be able to touch right foot. Then, bring body up again, using 8 counts, to starting position. B) Now kick right leg high, bring foot back in place; kick with left, bring back in place. Do this 8 times. C) Take a deep breath, hold one arm back and one arm forward, at shoulder level, and kick right leg, knee bent, up to chest. Do 8 times for each leg. D) Tilt body slightly back to right. Throw arms up toward ceiling as you do so and extend right leg out, so weight rests on heel. Change position to left side. Repeat over and over, going very fast. Relax and end up in Rest Position (explained in Warm-Ups for People Who Are on Their Feet All Day).

The Jogger

Jog around room, bringing knees up to chest, for 8 steps; then, jog 8 steps in place. Next, hop 8 steps around the room, making sure knee is high on each hop, and then do 8 hops in place. Alternate jogging and hopping until time is up and take a breather in Rest Position.

5

Figure Improvers/ Strengtheners

Any body looks better if everything is in proportion. And that's where firming and strengthening exercises come in. They can help smooth out bulges and make you appear trimmer and sleeker, even without losing weight. The Figure Improvers here do just that. The reason they work is this: when muscles aren't used, or are used very little, they foreshorten and fatty bulges form around them. As the muscles are strengthened and toned, the bulges disappear. Also, toned-up muscles take up less room than flabby, unused ones. Thus, you get a spot-reducing effect. In the case of the breast, which is made up of fatty tissue, the exercises develop the underlying pectoral muscles, so the bustline ends up looking firmer and more developed. However, exercises cannot do anything about changing bone structure (if it's bones, not flab, that give you your broad hips, that's a different problem).

To get the best results, check your Body Quiz, choose the exercises that apply to your trouble spots, and incorporate them into your daily workout. Aim for at least 7 minutes a day, more if you have the time. You should see results in three or four weeks, but keep in mind that *abdomen and waist will respond the most quickly, then hips, thighs, and buttocks, then breasts and calves.* Remember too, that the exercises in the other categories will be supplementing the effects of these Figure Improvers by toning and shaping your body in a general way.

For Abdomen

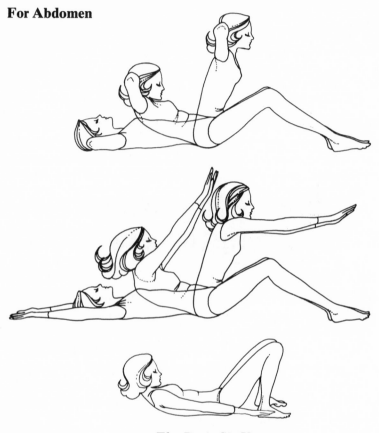

The Basic Sit-Up

Lie on back, knees bent, hands clasped together behind neck. Sit up with rounded back. Then lie down, keeping back rounded, and return to starting position. Do at least 5 times. If you cannot manage this sit-up, try either of these variations: lie on back, knees bent, arms overhead. Sit up with rounded back, chin to chest. Roll back to starting position slowly. Do 5 times. Or, lie on back, knees bent, arms at sides. Sit up with rounded back and then return to starting position, again with rounded back. Do 5 times.

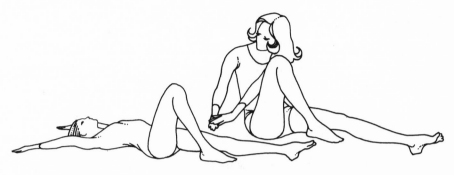

Sit-Up Twist (Advanced)

Lie on back, arms over head, left leg straight out and right leg bent. Sit up and twist to the right, bringing arms out past knee. Return to starting position. Do 4 times. Then, switch leg positions and do 4 more times.

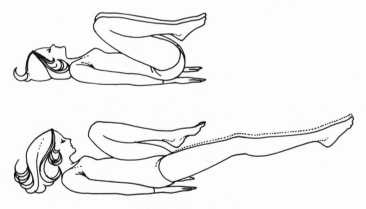

Leg Extension

Lie down on back with hands placed under bottom of buttocks, knees raised to chest. Stretch right leg forward, left leg forward, and return to starting position. Do 4 times.

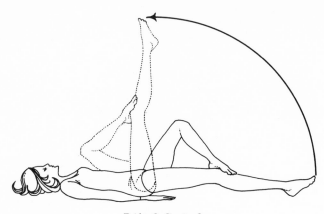

Lift & Switch

Lie down on back, hands under buttocks, right leg straight out on
floor and left foot resting on right knee. Raise both legs up as far
as you can, keeping their original foot-on-knee position. In mid-
air, switch position so right foot rests on left knee; then lower
to floor. Repeat, this time keeping right foot on left knee and
switching in mid-air to left foot on right knee. Do 4 times.

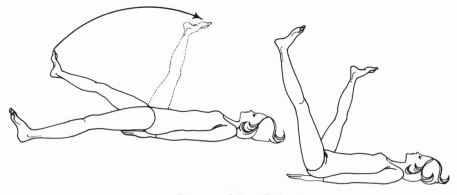

Diagonal Leg Lift

Lie on back, hands under buttocks, legs straight out and wide
apart. Raise right leg straight up, then left leg. Lower right leg,
then left. Do 4 times, but start with a different leg each time.
(Never raise both legs simultaneously.)

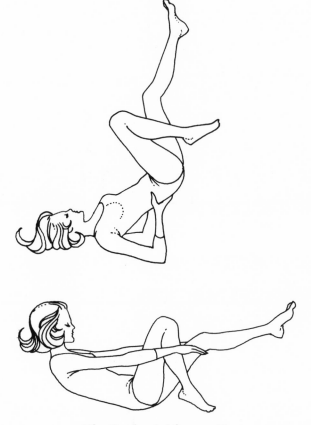

The Cycler (Advanced)

This is a variation of the popular "bicycle" exercise that you've probably done at one time or another. Do sequence fairly fast and try to keep rhythm even throughout. A) Lie on back with arms at sides. Raise legs upward, so they're perpendicular to floor, and pedal as you would a bicycle. Do for a count of 6; then sit up, still pedaling, to a count of 6. Go back down to starting position to another count of 6. B) Without interrupting rhythm, swing body upward and prop by holding waist with hands. Do this to a count of 6. Lower body back down to original position to a count of 6. Keep going for about 1 minute.

For Thighs, Hips, and Buttocks

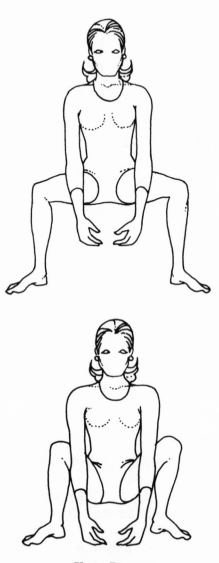

Knee Bounce

Stand up, feet apart, toes pointed outward, and keeping your back straight, bend knees and bounce 4 times, dipping body down below knees on each bounce. Raise up a bit and bounce 4 times again. Return to starting position. Repeat 4 times.

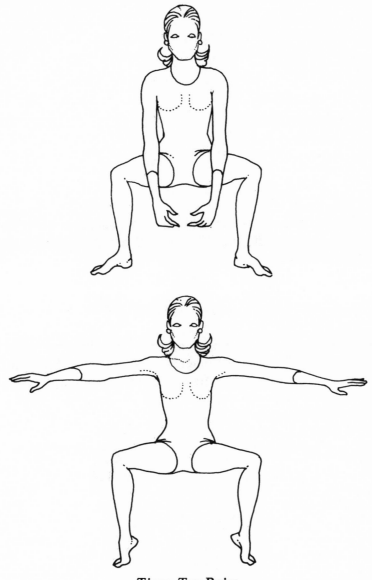

Tippy-Toe Raise

In same starting position as Knee Bounce, with bent knees, raise up on tiptoe and down on flat feet. Do 8 times. (Remember to keep bent-knee position throughout.) Shake out legs to release tension.

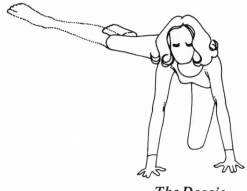

The Doggie

Go down on all fours. Raise right leg out to side, knee bent. Then extend leg out straight, bend again, and return to starting position. Do 6 times with each leg.

Inner Thigh Pull

Kneel, legs apart, back straight, and arms at sides. Pull knees in about one inch, using your inner thigh muscles, and hold for a count of 8. Release. If you are doing this properly, you should feel a definite tightness in inner thighs and buttocks. Repeat 6 times. (This is an isometric exercise.)

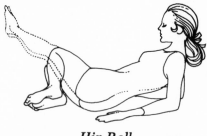

Hip Roll

From a sitting position, lean back on your forearms and bring bent knees up to chest. Roll to the right, twisting waist, and extend both legs out as you do so. Bend knees again, bring back to chest and roll to the left, again extending legs. Repeat, back and forth, 6 times on each side.

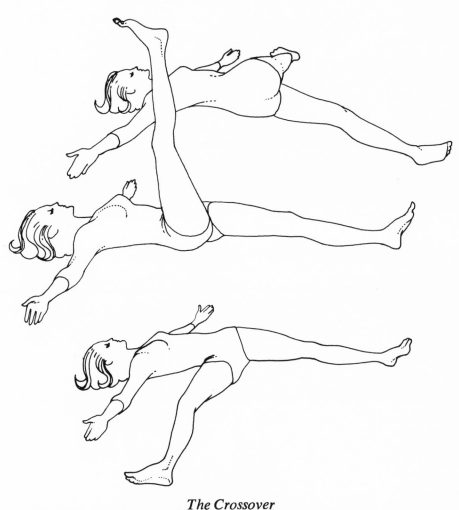

The Crossover

Lie on back, arms at shoulder level, legs straight. Raise right leg,
keeping knee straight, and cross it over body to left side and touch
foot to floor. Reverse direction, crossing to right side and touch
foot to floor. (Leg should be close to face during crossover.) Do
6 times with each leg.

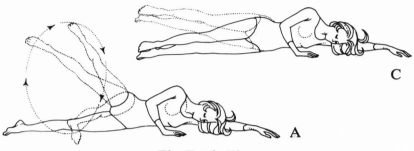

The Triple Threat

Lie down on left side with left arm extended up over head, right arm in front of chest for support. A) Circle upper leg at least 3 times in each direction. B) Next, move upper leg up and down as fast as possible. Repeat until tired, but do a minimum of 6 times. C) Now raise both legs up off floor; hold for a count of 3; then lower. Repeat at least 6 times. Turn over, and do exercises with left leg.

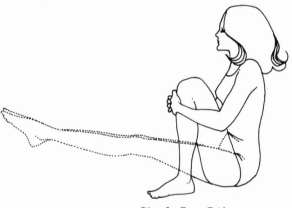

Single Leg Lift

Sit up with very straight back, right leg straight out, left leg bent. Grasp left knee close to body, so that chest touches leg. Without moving body, lift right leg up off floor as far as you can, and return to floor. Then lift again, move out to the side of body, and touch floor; lift once more, bring back in front of body, and touch floor. (Not illustrated.) Repeat 6 times; then switch leg positions and do 6 times with left leg.

For Waist

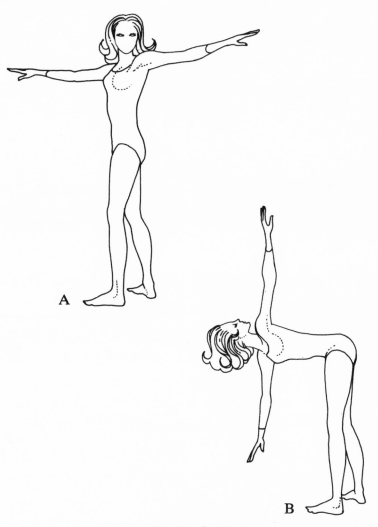

The Studio Twist

A) Stand up, legs apart, arms out at shoulder level. Twist body from side to side, keeping legs in stationary position. Do 10 times. B) Bend down, from hips, with a flat back. Twist from side to side, so that one arm points to the floor and one to ceiling. Repeat 10 times.

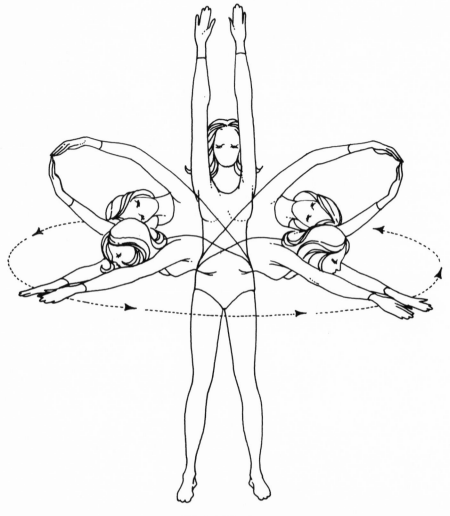

Waist Circles

Stand up, feet apart, arms pointed to ceiling. Bend from waist and stretch to right, then move to center, then to left side. Come up to starting position. Reverse direction. Repeat 10 times.

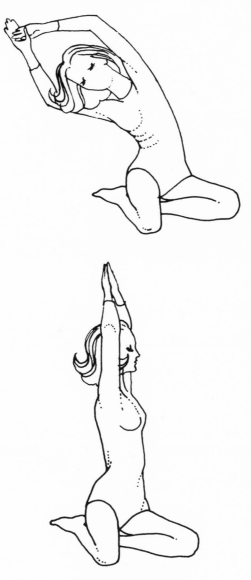

The Body Twister

Sit down with both legs tucked under body and pointing to one side. Raise arms over head and bend toward feet; then sit up straight and twist back and away from feet. Return to starting position. Do 5 times with legs to one side, 5 times to other side.

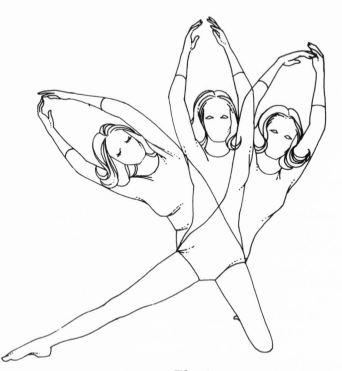

The Arc

Kneel on left knee, right leg extended out to side, and arms raised up toward ceiling. Bend slowly to right side, then stretch away from right leg and bend down to opposite side. Do 3 times, then switch leg positions and do 3 times more.

For Bust and Upper Arms

Arm Circles

Standing or sitting, hold arms out at shoulder level. Turn arms under from shoulder and face palms toward ceiling. (If you are doing this properly, you should feel a tenseness in your upper arms already.) Circle forward 10 times, then circle backward 10 times.

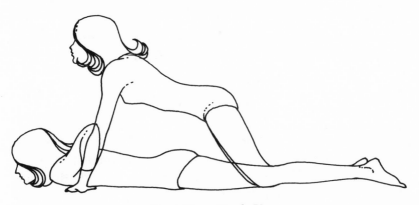

Bent Knee Push-Up

Lie on stomach, hands on floor near shoulders, elbows bent. Push body up off floor, using arm muscles to do so, until you are in a kneeling position. Return to starting position. Repeat 10 times.

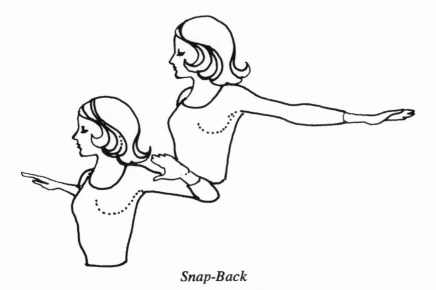

Snap-Back

Sitting or standing, hold arms out at shoulder level and bend elbows. Snap elbows back; return to starting position. Then, swing arms straight back and return to starting position. Repeat 8 times.

The Pectoral Snap

Standing or sitting, grasp forearms with hands and push skin of forearms toward elbows. Relax. Repeat 25 times, fast.

Breast Stroke

Sitting or standing, hold arms out at shoulder level and bend elbows. Press palms together and point forward. Stretch arms forward and out in a fluid motion, and then swing to back. Return to starting position. Repeat 10 times.

For Calves

These exercises will help develop the calf muscles and give legs a prettier, shapelier look.

Tiptoe Lift

Stand up straight and slowly rise up on tiptoes. Hold for a count of 6; return to flat foot position. Repeat 20 times.

One Foot Stance

Stand up straight and hold onto back of chair with one hand. Raise up on one foot to tiptoe position, and hold other leg slightly above floor for a count of 6. Switch to other leg in tiptoe position. Do 6 times on each leg.

6

Stamina Build-Ups

Fact: You can have a good shape, but not necessarily be in good shape. Fact: The proper exercise can put you in better shape by increasing your endurance. How? By doing aerobic exercises, which force you to take in more oxygen and thereby strengthen the heart and improve lung function. And when your cardio-pulmonary efficiency increases, your system's ability to deliver oxygen-bearing blood to your whole body improves. Once this happens, you have more energy (since oxygen is fuel for energy), and your capacity for activity increases. And, as a working woman, you *know* how important that is! Done regularly, aerobic exercises will even help reduce fatigue, improve general health, and aid in sleeping better—all because you won't require as many breaths to get the needed amount of oxygen, so, as a result, your heart and lungs won't have to work as hard.

The Stamina Build-Ups here are all aerobic. They should be done as fast as possible, by everyone, at least a few times a week. If you tend to tire very easily, do approximately 30 minutes' worth a week. Keep in mind that the Warm-Ups are also aerobic and alternate them with the Stamina Build-Ups for variety.

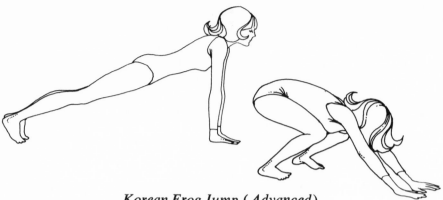

Korean Frog Jump (Advanced)

Go down on all fours and stretch body out above floor so that weight is balanced on hands and toes. Jump forward so that feet end up close to hands and press heels down. Jump back to starting position. Repeat 10 times, moving as fast as possible.

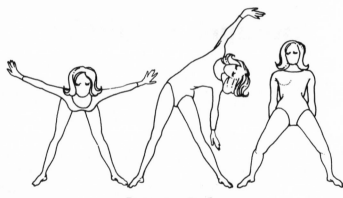

Bouncing Body

Stand up, legs apart, arms straight out at shoulder level. A) Bend forward, flat back (back parallel to floor), and bounce up and down 8 times. B) Return to starting position and bounce to the left 8 times, with your right arm curving overhead and left arm hanging down at your side. Repeat 8 times to the right. C) Return to starting position and bounce backward by bending knees and tilting pelvis forward. Keep arms at sides. Do 8 times. Repeat entire series again, this time doing 4 bounces. Then repeat, doing 2 bounces, then 1 bounce.

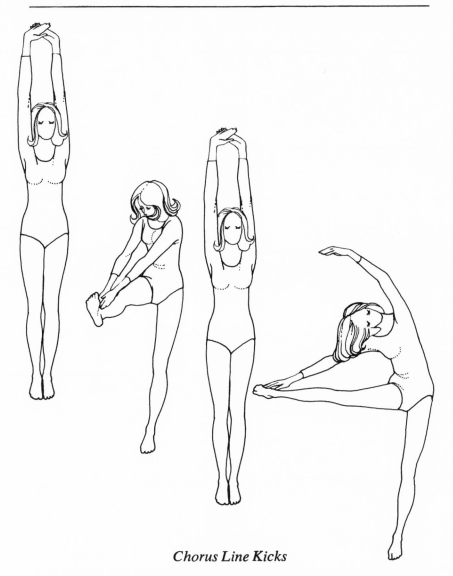

Chorus Line Kicks

A) Stand up straight, arms over head. Bend from waist and at the same time, bring right leg up. Try to touch arm to leg. Return to starting position. Switch to left leg. Repeat at least 8 times for each leg and do entire sequence very fast. B) In the same starting position, bend sideways to the right and kick right leg up. Try to touch arm to leg. Return to starting position. Repeat 8 times on each side.

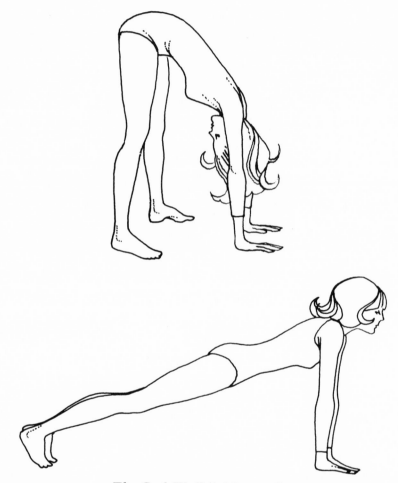

The Crab Walk (Advanced)

From a standing position, bend down and place hands flat on floor. Trying to keep legs as straight as possible, walk forward on hands until body is almost parallel with floor. Pause and walk backward on hands until they meet feet. Raise up to standing position. Repeat 4 times. (If you cannot keep legs absolutely straight, do with slightly bent knees.)

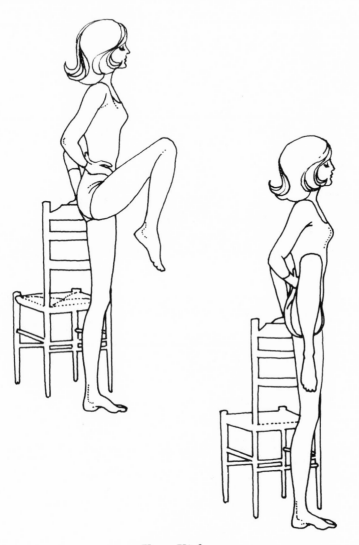

Knee Kicker

Stand up and hold onto a chair with left hand for support. Bring right knee up to chest 4 times. Then, kick right leg out to the side 4 times, bringing it out from the hip and then in to the front of body. Repeat this out-to-the-side, in-to-the-front motion 4 times. Switch to other leg and repeat entire sequence 4 times for 1 minute.

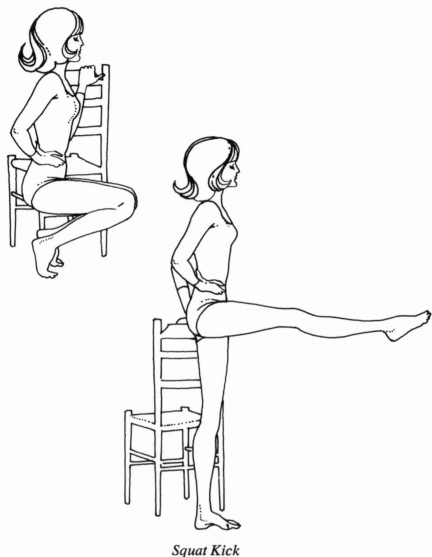

Squat Kick

Stand up straight, hold onto the back of a chair with left hand, place right hand on waist. Lower body into a squat position, then come up quickly, kicking right leg as high as possible when you do so. Repeat 5 times. Then, switch position, and kick with left leg.

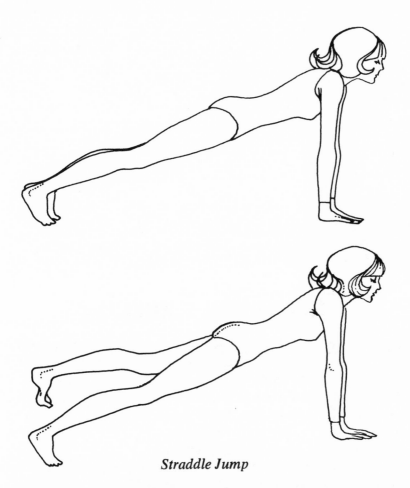

Straddle Jump

Go down on all fours and stretch body out above floor so that weight is balanced on hands and toes. Jump and open legs wide; jump again, this time bringing them back together. Do very fast for at least 10 times.

7

Flexibility Exercises

Okay. So you've worked on exercises to trim down those bulges, build up your stamina, strengthen weak muscles—what next? Flexibility. Or, in other words, a graceful, supple body. And if that doesn't sound like much, consider this: if you're supple you automatically look younger because you move better; you'll hold yourself more confidently because good flexibility improves posture (extremely important to your working image); you're less apt to stumble because your muscles are elastic, and if you do, there's less likelihood that you'll hurt yourself.

But how do you increase your flexibility? By doing the exercises here. They're designed to stretch the ligaments of your joints in all directions to their fullest potential and they work on increasing the elasticity of the muscles. Done on a regular basis, they'll help you to become more limber and adaptable to all kinds of movements. Do all of them *slowly*. The idea is to aim for a flowing, rhythmic movement. If flexibility is a prime problem (check your Body Quiz), do 2 or 3 minutes of them daily, and switch the various exercises around, so you cover the whole program. If not, include a few minutes of them a week, when you have the time, to insure a supple body.

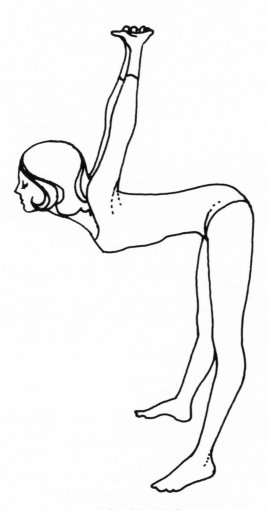

Shoulder Pull

Stand up straight, legs apart, arms down, and hands clasped behind back. Pull shoulder blades together, bend forward from the
hips, keeping back straight, and raise arms up as far as possible.
Return to starting position. Do 5 times. (Good for back and
shoulder flexibility, as well as hamstrings, which are the back
thigh muscles.)

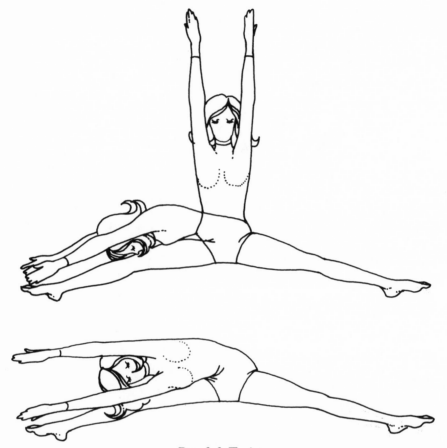

Bend & Twist

Sit down on floor, back straight, legs apart, and arms straight above your head. Bend body toward your right foot and try to touch head to right knee. Bounce 3 times. Then, twist toward the inside of your leg, so that right side is about parallel to right leg. Bounce 3 times. Return to starting position. Alternate sides and do 5 times on each side. (Good for back, hamstring, and waist flexibility.)

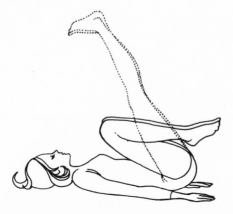

Heel Stretch

Lie on back, arms at sides, knees to chest. Flex ankles and straighten legs out, keeping ankles flexed as you do so. (Movement should be such that heels look as if they are being pushed toward ceiling.) Return to starting position. Do 5 times. (Good for hamstring flexibility.)

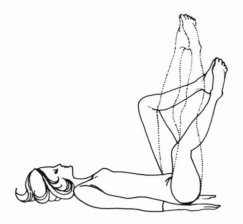

Sole Clapper

Lie on back, arms at sides, legs up in air and soles of feet pressed together. Stretch legs up as far as possible, keeping soles together. Return to starting position. Do 5 times. (Good for inner thigh and ankle flexibility.)

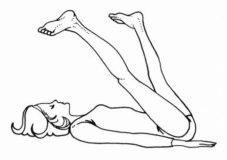

Foot Thrust

Lie on back, knees to chest, ankles flexed. Thrust feet away from each other in opposite directions. Hold and bounce 3 times. Return to starting position. Do 5 times. (Good for inner thigh flexibility.)

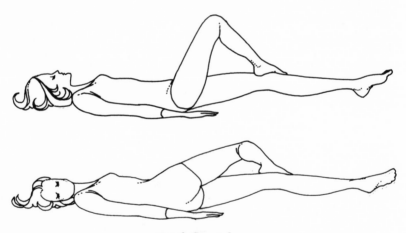

Back Stretcher

Lie flat on back, arms at sides, with right foot on left knee. Bend over to the left, keeping shoulders on floor and easing right leg over slowly, so you feel a stretch in your waist area. Face should look toward right (away from direction of stretch) as you do this. Return to starting position. Switch leg positions and move toward right. Continue alternating, 10 times on each side. (Good for back flexibility.)

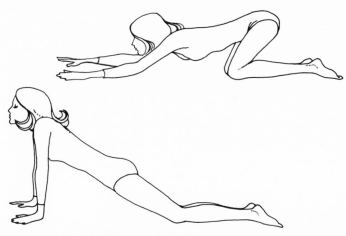

Pectoral Stretch

Get down on knees, arms out in front of you, palms on floor, so that body is at a slant. Bounce shoulders 3 times, making sure you don't bend elbows. (If you are doing this correctly, you'll feel the stretch in your pectorals.) Then, slowly lift body forward, keeping arms straight, so legs end up straight out on floor and body is supported by arms. Hold for a count of 3. Return to starting position. Do 5 times. (Good for pectoral and shoulder flexibility.)

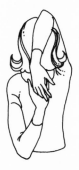

The Zipper Pull

Sitting or standing, reach right arm over right shoulder and bring your left arm toward your back and stretch it upward. Try to touch hands. Switch arm positions. Do 5 times in each position. (Good for shoulder flexibility.)

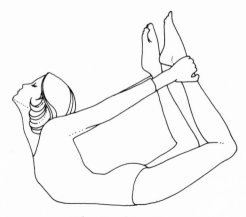

The Rocking Horse

Lie on stomach, bend knees, and grasp ankles with hands. Pull feet away from body, so knees are lifted off the floor. Hold for a count of 3. Return to starting position. Do 5 times. As you get better, try to achieve a smooth rocking motion. (Good for thigh and torso flexibility.)

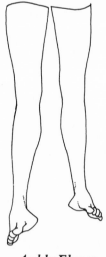

Ankle Flexer

Walk 4 steps on the outside of your feet; relax. Repeat, continuing for 30 seconds to 1 minute. (Good for ankle and foot flexibility.)

8

Tension Releasers

If your solution to a hard day at work is to take a run around the block, hop on a bike, or scrub the floor, you're really not doing yourself as much good as you could. Although any of these activities might help you cool off, chances are you're still tight and anxious inside. What you should do are slow, easy exercises to stretch out and ease those muscles that have contracted during the day. Unlike the run around the block (which contracts muscles), this will relax your muscles and help prevent the tightness and spasms that lead to headaches, backaches, and the like. That's also why any regular exercise routine that includes lots of stretching exercises, like the ones in this book, is one of the best antidotes to tension.

The exercises in this chapter, done in the sequence explained, make up a good 5-minute Tension Release program. Use it by itself whenever you feel particularly tense or irritable, or as a prelude to your regular routine. Otherwise, include the Tension Releasers that apply to your personal trouble spots (shoulders, neck, back, whatever) in your daily workout immediately after your warm-ups. By doing this, you'll help to ward off greater tension because you'll be taking care of normal, everyday tension on a regular basis.

The Prime Unwinder

Lie down, flat on back, arms at sides. Close eyes. Breathe deeply, in and out, for a count of 20. Then, rotate right ankle; relax. Rotate left ankle; relax. Tighten right thigh; relax. Tighten left thigh; relax. Stomach. Buttocks. Right arm. Left arm. Screw up face and then un-tense. Let body go totally limp; then tighten, go limp again. Breathe deeply, inhaling through nose and exhaling through mouth. This exercise should take 1 minute. (Relaxes entire body.)

Arm Flapper

Lie down, flat on back, arms at sides, legs straight. Raise right arm so hand points toward ceiling; let drop. Repeat with left arm. Continue alternating arms, and do 3 times for each arm. (Relaxes arm muscles.)

Head Raise

Lie down, flat on back, arms at sides, legs straight. Raise head so that chin comes up to touch chest. Lower head back to floor. Do 5 times. (Stretches back of neck muscles, and also strengthens stomach muscles.)

Slow Rocker

Lie down on back, knees to chest, and hug knees to body. Keeping head on floor, rock gently for 30 seconds to 1 minute. (Relieves lower back tension.)

Leg Stretcher

Lie on left side with left arm straight and under head, right arm in front of chest for support. Bring right knee to chest, then return to starting position. Repeat 5 times. Then roll over to other side and do 5 times with left leg. (Relaxes leg muscles.)

Stomach Pelvic Tilt

Lie on stomach and rest head on crossed arms. Pull stomach off the floor and contract buttocks at the same time. Hold for a count of 5. Relax. Do 5 times.

Elbow Circles

Sit up in a crosslegged position, back straight. Put fingertips on shoulder caps and rotate elbows backward in a big circle. Pause. Do 3 times, always pausing between circles; then, reverse direction, and do 3 forward circles. (Relaxes tense shoulders and neck muscles.)

Head Roll

Still sitting crosslegged, drop chin to right shoulder; lift, and drop to left shoulder. Return to starting position. Do 3 times. (Relaxes neck muscles.)

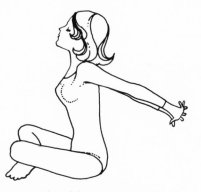

Shoulder Loosener

In same position, interlock fingers behind back and rest palms on floor. Pull shoulders together by lifting and stretching arms upward. Drop arms and slump forward. Return to starting position and do 5 times. (Eases shoulder tension.)

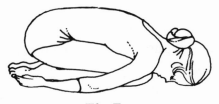

The Fetus

Go into a fetal position by kneeling, with derriere resting on
heels and placing arms at side of body and head on floor. Let
every muscle in your body, including face, go absolutely limp.
Hold for 30 seconds to 1 minute. (Good overall relaxer.)

9

Posture/Balance Fixers

No exercise program is complete without some mention of posture and coordination. These two important aspects can make or break your overall appearance. In addition, poor posture can lead to back problems, shoulder tension (just think what is happening to your body when you slump over the typewriter), or a protruding stomach. It also makes you look older and less confident. Poor balance can cause you to stumble (which is the last thing you want to do when entering a meeting), hinder you in sports, and may eventually bring on a bad fall.

Now, not everyone has these problems (check your Body Quiz), but if you do, you must include the necessary exercises in your program to correct them. Since both good posture and good balance depend on proper alignment and weight centering, exercises for both are included here. Do both sets, or just one, depending on your individual needs, at least 3 times a week. The nice thing about this mini-program is that the basic posture exercises—the Pelvic Tilt and the Box Stackup—can be done quickly and easily in most any place at all. And once you've got that alignment down pat, your balance will also improve.

For Posture

In order to have, and sustain, correct posture, all the skeletal muscles must be in good shape. That's why you need a total exercise program. However, if your posture is particularly bad, the exercises here will help. Try to do them a few times a week. Also, keep the Posture Reminders in mind and use them a few times a day or whenever you think about it. You'll be surprised at how a little checking up on yourself can improve your posture, quickly and easily.

Basic Pelvic Tilt

Lie on back, knees bent, feet on floor. Put one hand on lower abdomen, the other under small of back. Contract buttock muscles. (You should feel spine press against hand at this point.) Relax. Contract abdominal muscles. (The hand on your abdomen should sink down at this point.) Do not hold breath. Then, do both contractions together. Repeat over and over. As you get the feel of this, you'll no longer need to place your hands this way and can just keep them at your sides. Practice the Pelvic Tilt standing up as well as lying down on stomach and back.

The Box Stackup

Stand sideways in front of a full-length mirror and imagine that your body is made up of four boxes—one each for your head, upper torso, lower torso, and legs. Boxes should be aligned as shown in sketch. If your boxes are off, straighten up like this:

a) distribute weight evenly between balls and heels of feet
b) do Pelvic Tilt by contracting buttocks and abdomen (this will straighten lower spine)
c) pull shoulder blades toward spine (do not roll *shoulders* back —that only gives a military stance)
d) drop shoulders as low as possible
e) hold chin parallel to floor
f) imagine that a string is pulling you up from the center of your head

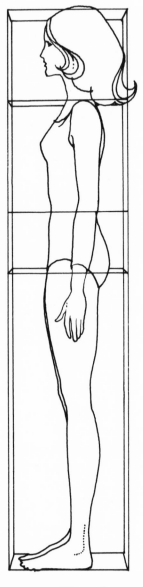

Once you are in the correct position, slump. Repeat Box Stackup at least 3 times. Note: Don't be surprised if you feel as if you are tipping forward. The position is correct; you are just not used to it. After continued practice, correct posture alignment will come naturally.

Back Strengthener Series

Before you begin this series of exercises, do the Body Stretch and the Leg Stretch from the Warm-Ups chapter.

A) Lie on stomach, arms next to ears and straight out above head. Slowly raise your right arm, left leg, and head all at once, and up as far as possible. Then, lower slowly. Next, raise left arm, right leg, and head in the same way, and then lower. Do 4 times with each arm and leg. B) In the same position, slowly raise both arms and both legs up at once. Lower back to starting position. Repeat 4 times. C) In the same starting position, do the Stomach Pelvic Tilt, where you pull stomach off the floor and contract buttock muscles at the same time. Hold. Relax. Do 4 times. D) Still in same starting position, raise upper body (head, shoulders, chest) off floor and bring arms down to sides of body. Relax and lower body. Then, raise upper body again, bring arms up and back to starting position. Relax and lower body. Do 4 times. E) Still on stomach, put arms at sides of body. Press arms into floor and raise both legs upward from the hip. Return to starting position. Do 4 times.

Posture Reminders

Sitting Check

Lift ribcage high and pull shoulder blades together. Do not push shoulders back—it is your shoulder *blades* that must be close to spine.

Wake-Up Check

Since many women sleep on their sides in a semi-fetal position, this exercise is based on that position. To do, stay on side, but straighten legs out; then do Pelvic Tilt (pull abdomen in, contract buttocks) and hold. Simultaneously pull shoulders back and down, pull head up, and place top arm on thigh. Slump. Repeat once more. (If you sleep on stomach or back, just roll over to side and then do exercise.)

Walking Check

As you're walking along, roll weight from heel forward to ball of foot until you feel as if you're tilted forward. At the same time, do the Pelvic Tilt (pull abdomen in, contract buttocks). Continue rolling weight back and forth from heel to ball of foot as you take each step.

For Balance

If you stumble a lot or feel generally "uncoordinated," you might try these exercises. They'll help improve your balance and coordination by centering your weight properly. They're also worthwhile if you participate in sports where you need a good sense of balance. Start by doing the Box Stackup (page 000) for proper alignment, then tighten leg and stomach muscles and begin.

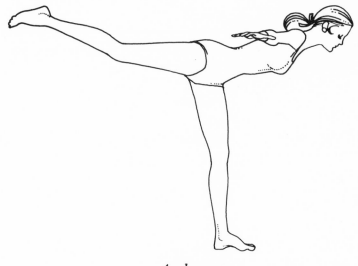

Arabesque

Stand up straight, arms out at shoulder level. Bend forward and raise one leg out straight behind you, trying to get it parallel to floor. (If you stare at one spot in front of you, it helps.) Return to starting position. Alternate legs and do 4 times on each leg.

The Teeter-Totter

Stand up straight, tighten stomach muscles, and center weight over one leg. Raise the other leg, bending knee as you do so. Hold position for a count of 5. Return to starting position. Center weight on other leg. Alternate back and forth, 4 times on each leg. As you get better, do with closed eyes. (The first few times you do this exercise with closed eyes, stand near a wall that you can grab onto just in case you falter.)

Leg Circles

Stand up straight, arms at sides. Raise one leg off the floor, as high as possible, and keeping leg straight, move it in a semi-circle from front to side to back; then reverse direction. Return to starting position. Alternate legs and do 4 times on each leg.

Tiptoe Stretcher

Stand up straight, arms at sides. Raise up on tiptoes. Balance on one foot for a count of 5. Return other foot to floor and relax tiptoe position. Do 4 times on each leg, alternating legs.

10

Cool-Offs

After any exercise routine, your muscles are in an excited, warmed-up state and need to be relaxed. And the way to do that is not to jump into the shower or lie down on the bed, but to do a couple more minutes of exercising. The reason? By finishing off your workout with some slow and easy movements, you give your system a chance to return to normal. Cool-Offs will slow down your blood circulation, relax your muscles, and wind down your nerves. If you eliminate them, you subject your body to unnecessary stress because it will have no transition period in which to normalize gradually.

There are three different Cool-Off series here. You can do any one you like to finish off your exercises depending on your mood. Each of them should be done for about 2 minutes, however, so time yourself. If you finish too quickly you are not moving slowly enough.

The Windmill

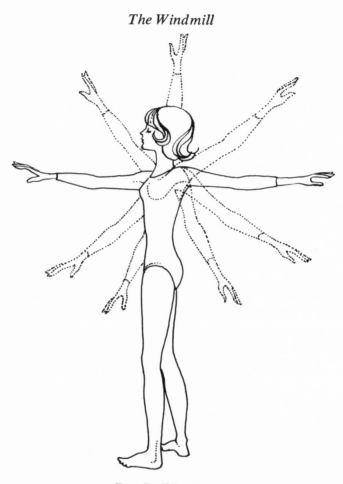

Rag Doll Series

Stand up straight, arms at sides. Swing right leg back and forth
a few times, gradually slowing pace, until leg goes limp. Repeat
with left leg. Then, circle right arm around and around, reversing
direction once, and let drop loosely. Repeat with left arm. Drop
head and let torso hang down. Hold for a few counts. Finish by
bringing torso up slowly, vertebra by vertebra, until you stand up
straight.

Sit-Down Coolers

The following exercises should be done in the sequence explained here. A) Sit crosslegged, back straight, hands interlocked and in lap. Bring arms up over head and as far back as possible, stretching the upper part of your body as you do so. Hold this position and bounce 6 times. Return to starting position. Repeat 6 times. B) Unclasp hands and raise arms straight over head. Pull ribcage out of waist and stretch right side up to ceiling. Return to starting position. Stretch left side up to ceiling. (When you do this, you should feel the pull in your waist.) Do 6 times on each side. C) Still sitting, lean back on left elbow, and extend left leg out straight on floor. Grasp right heel from inside with right hand and stretch leg upward as far as it can go. (Try to get it as straight as possible.) Return to starting position. Do 6 times.

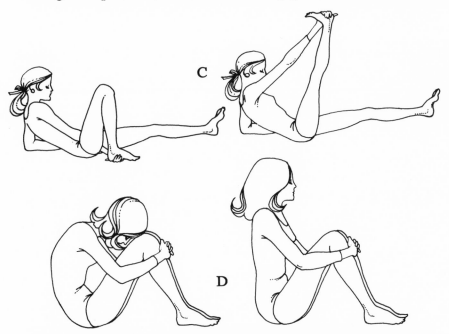

Then, switch position, and do 6 times with left leg. D) Sit up with bent knees, arms around legs and head resting on knees. Starting from the base of your spine, slowly straighten up and raise head, until you are in perfect posture. Then, slump and return to starting position. Repeat 6 times.

Lazy Woman's Cool-Offs

Lie down on right side, right arm under head, left arm on thigh. Raise left arm slowly up and toward head until it touches other hand and stretch from fingertips to toes. Return to starting position. Do 4 times, then turn over, and do 4 times on left side. Next, roll over onto back, relax, and inhale and exhale deeply. Continue deep breathing for 30 seconds, or until 2 minutes are up.

11

Specialty Exercises

Even though this whole exercise program is geared to a total body system, there are going to be times when your priorities change and your basic exercise routine won't meet your new demands. For instance, what exercises will help you get in shape for tennis, for jogging, for skiing? Or alleviate bad menstrual cramps? This chapter will tell you. It's devoted to specific situations like pre-sport preparation and cramps and post-natal needs.

All of the Specialty Exercises are supplementary to your regular program. The Menstrual Soothers and Post-Natal Shape-Up are to be done instead of it; the pre-sport programs in addition to it. Since the Pre-Tennis and Pre-Ski workouts do take up a fair chunk of time—10 minutes—you might want to concentrate on them for a while and cut down your regular routine somewhat. For example, do them 3 times a week; your normal program the other 4 days. The Jogging Curriculum takes up much less time and can be done right along with your other exercises.

Pre-Ski Workout

The following exercises should be preceded by 3 minutes of

73

Warm-Ups for a good get-in-shape-for-ski-season routine. The entire workout should be done in the sequence explained here and should take 10 minutes.

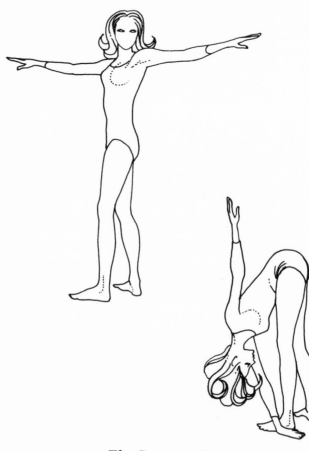

The Crossover Twist

Stand up, arms at shoulder level, legs wide apart. Twist and bend, so that right hand touches left heel, and bounce a few times. Switch, and touch left hand to right heel and bounce. Do 10 times on each side. Return to starting position. (This improves overall flexibility and increases elasticity of waist.)

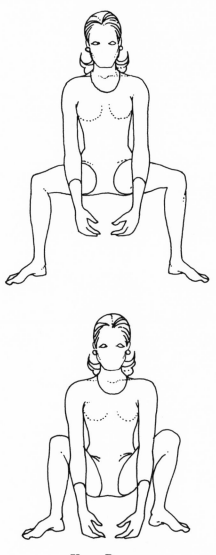

Knee Bounce

Still standing up, bend knees and bounce deep down below knee level 4 times. Straighten up and return to starting position. Do 10 times. Shake out legs to relieve tension. (This exercise strengthens thighs.)

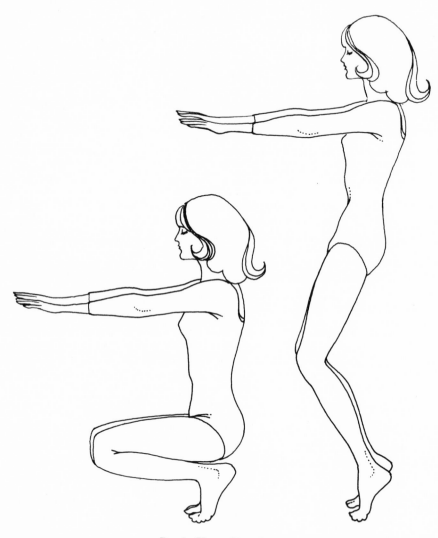

Basic Knee Bend

Stand up straight, arms straight out in front of body. Bend knees and slowly lower body, keeping a straight back, until thighs are parallel with floor. Then, push pelvis forward as you come back up to starting position. Do 10 times. (This helps strengthen thighs and back.)

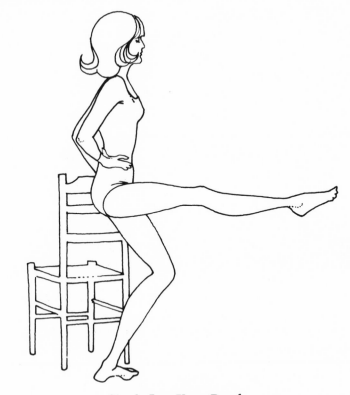

Single Leg Knee Bend

Stand up straight, one hand on chair for support, other hand on waist. With one leg raised above floor, bend other knee and slowly lower body down as far as possible. Return to starting position. Do 10 times on each leg. If it is too difficult, stand between two chairs and hold onto each for support. (This also helps to strengthen thighs and back and improves balance.)

Forward Lean

Stand on a telephone book, so that the back half of your feet hang over it. Holding arms straight out in front of you, bend knees, press heels toward floor, and lower body until you are in a forward lean position and bounce 3 times. Straighten up slowly. Repeat 10 times. (This improves flexibility of ankles.)

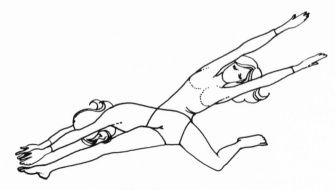

The Wipeout

Sit down, back straight, right leg straight out in front of you, left leg turned toward back and bent at knee. Bend body slowly forward in the direction of your straight leg and try to touch your head to your knee. Return to starting position. Bend slowly sideways toward other knee. Return to starting position. Do 3 times, then switch leg positions, and do 3 more times. (This improves flexibility of entire body.)

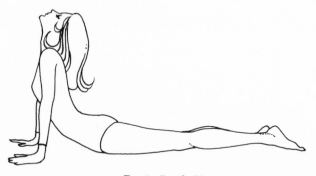

Basic Push-Up

Lie on stomach, hands near head, elbows bent outward. Push upper part of body up, leaving legs on floor. Return to starting position. Do 10 times.

Finish up with 10 Basic Sit-Ups (Chapter 5—Figure Improvers/Strengtheners) and the Bouncing Body exercise (Chapter 6—Stamina Build-Ups).

Pre-Tennis Routine

Like the Pre-Ski workout, the following exercises should be preceded by 3 minutes of Warm-Ups. Do in the sequence explained here for a terrific 10-minute tennis shape-up.

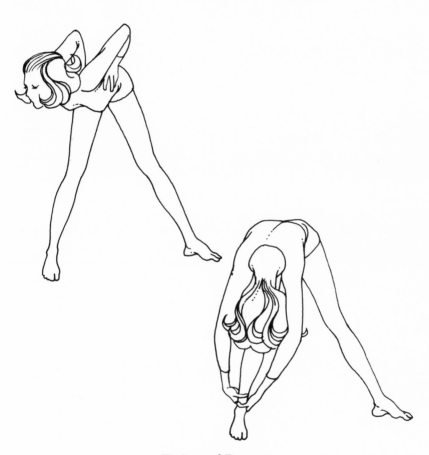

Twist and Bounce

Stand up straight, legs wide apart, hands on waist. Twist and bend over right leg, keeping back straight, and bounce up and down 4 times. Then, with a rounded back, grasp right ankle, touch head to knee, and bounce 4 times. Return to starting position. Repeat on other side. Next, do 2 bounces in each position, then 1 bounce. (This improves flexibility and stamina.)

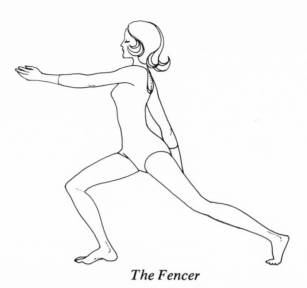

The Fencer

Stand up straight, feet together, arms at sides. Lunge forward on right leg, bringing left arm forward as you do so. Return to starting position. Do 5 times with each leg. (This increases leg strength and improves stroke movement.)

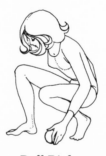

Ball Pickup

Stand up straight, arms at sides. Bend knees way down and reach toward floor as though you were picking up a ball with your left hand. Straighten up, take a forward step, and then bend down again, and pick up the "ball" with your right hand. Continue stepping around room and picking up "ball" for 30 seconds. (This improves coordination and flexibility and strengthens legs.)

Basic Push-Up

(See explanation in Pre-Ski Workout p. 73–74.)

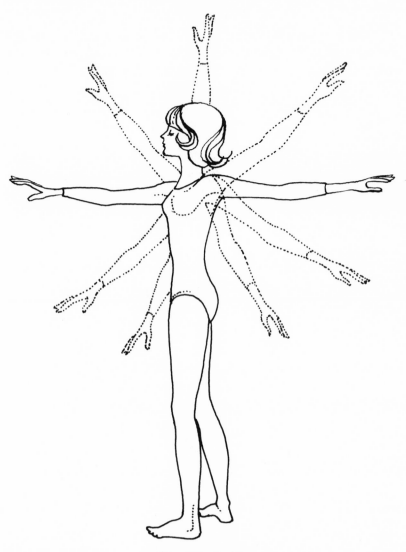

The Windmill

Stand up straight and swing both arms in fast circles, going backward, then forward, for 30 seconds. Don't cheat—make sure arms go *back*. (This limbers up arms and helps overhead stroke.)

Basic Sit-Up

Finish up with 10 Basic Sit-Ups (Chapter 5—Figure Improvers/Strengtheners).

The following two exercises can be done as part of the Pre-Tennis routine, or whenever you have time. Both can be done sitting or standing, and both strengthen wrists and forearms.

Hand Squeeze

With an old tennis ball in each hand, stretch arms out at shoulder level and squeeze balls hard; then relax. Do at least 20 times.

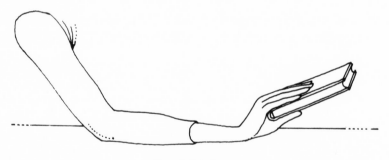

Book Pickup

Holding a book in hand, rest your forearm on a table or counter. Then, moving only your wrist, raise the book up and hold for a count of 5. Put book down; relax. Do 5 times. (This helps strengthen forearm.)

Jogging Curriculum

If you plan on starting a jogging program, it's a good idea to shape up first with a series of exercises that will build up your stamina and strengthen your muscles, especially those in calves and thighs. Below, you'll find a listing of exercises that are particularly helpful. Try to start doing them about 2 weeks before you begin jogging. They only take 6 or 7 minutes, including Warm-Ups, and so can be incorporated easily into your regular routine. Then, once you start jogging, do the Before and After workouts.

Pre-Jogging Shapers

Start by doing the Basic Body Relaxer (Chapter 4) for 1 minute and follow it with the Warm-Ups of your choice. Then, lie down and do some Basic Sit-Ups. Begin with at least 5 and work up to 15. This will help strengthen the abdomen. Next, do 10 Diagonal Leg Lifts (both, Chapter 5—Figure Improvers) to strengthen your diagonal stomach muscles—important in running. Turn over onto stomach and do the Back Strengtheners (Chapter 9—Posture/Balance Fixers). Stand up and do the Tippy-Toe Raise (Chapter 5—a calf and thigh strengthener). For stamina, do the Squat Kick (Chapter 6—Stamina Build-Ups). (If you are doing these exercises by themselves, and not as part of your regular routine, finish up with 2 minutes of the Cool-Offs of your choice —Chapter 10.)

Before Jogging

Warm up with the Bouncing Body (Chapter 6—Stamina Build-Ups) to help increase endurance. Then, do this "Goose Step." Still in standing position, kick up high with right leg, step forward; kick up high with left leg, step forward. Do all around the room for about 1 minute. Finish with Rest Position (Chapter 4—Warm-Ups).

After Jogging

While muscles are still in a warmed-up, excited state, do the following stretches: A) Stand up, cross feet at ankles, and keeping knees straight, bend over and try to touch floor with hands. Return to starting position. Do 5 times. B) Still standing up, put one heel on the seat of a chair and bend over, trying to touch head to other knee. Do 3 times. Then, switch legs and do 3 more times. C) Next, lie down on back and do the Heel Stretch and the Rocking Horse (both, Chapter 7—Flexibility Exercises).

Menstrual Soothers

The following exercises may be helpful if you suffer from menstrual cramps, because they stretch the pelvic area and thus help the uterus to relax. Since it is usually the contracted muscles of the uterus that cause cramps, this relaxation effect often helps the cramps to subside. Do the exercises very slowly, and stop at once if cramps get worse.

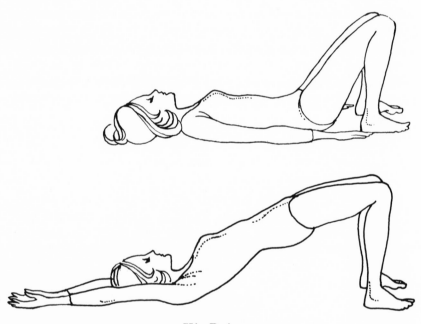

Hip Raise

Lie down on back, arms at sides, knees bent, feet on floor. Contract buttocks, bring arms up over head, and lift hips to a count of 5. Stretch. Go back down to a count of 5, so that small of back hits floor first, and buttocks hit floor last. Repeat 5 times.

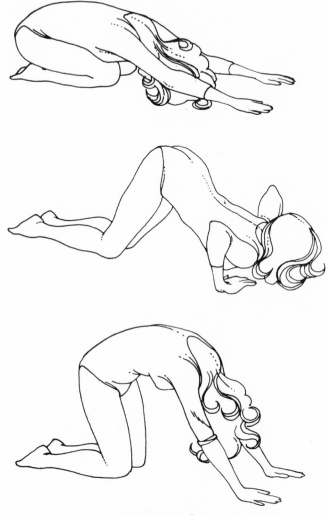

Chin Crawler

Sit back on heels, knees apart, chin near to floor and arms straight out in front of you with hands on floor. Pretend you are licking up chocolate and slowly bring chin forward, bending elbows as you do so, until head is between hands. Raise up slowly with a rounded back, pulling your stomach in, and go back down to starting position. Do 5 times.

Post-Natal Shape-Up

The following exercises are especially designed not to put too much stress on your body. Done in the sequence explained here, they will take about 5 minutes and will help firm flabby abdominal muscles and strengthen back muscles. Do them slowly and if you feel any discomfort, stop the exercise at once. To be on the safe side, check with your doctor before you begin this program.

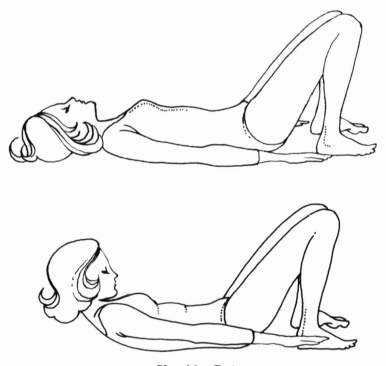

Shoulder Raise

Lie on back, knees bent, feet on floor, arms at sides. Raise head and shoulders slowly off the floor and hold for a count of 10. Return to starting position. Do 5 times. Gradually work up to a point where you actually can sit up. This may take a while, so don't push it—go at your own pace, but try a bit harder each time.

Easy Leg Lift

Lie on back, knees bent to chest, arms at sides. Extend one leg straight above the floor and hold for a count of 4. Return to starting position. Extend other leg and hold for a count of 4. Continue alternating legs and do 4 times with each leg.

Basic Pelvic Tilt

Lie on back, knees bent, feet on floor. Contract buttocks, and at the same time, pull lower abdomen in without holding breath. Hold for a count of 4 and relax. (If you are doing this properly, the small of your back should be pressed against the floor when you contract. (For a fuller explanation, see Chapter 9—Posture/ Balance Fixers.) Do 4 times.

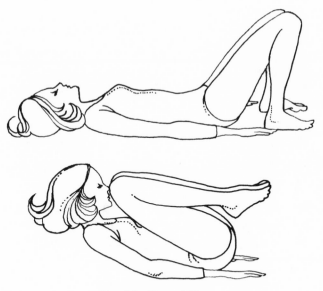

Double Knee Kiss

Lie on back, knees bent, feet on floor, arms at sides. Keeping arms on the floor, bring upper body forward and knees backward until knees touch nose. Hold. Return to starting position. Do 4 times.

Leg Extender

Lie down, arms at sides, knees bent and up on chest. Extend right leg up toward ceiling and flex ankle. Bring back to starting position. Do with left leg. Continue alternating legs and do 4 times with each leg.

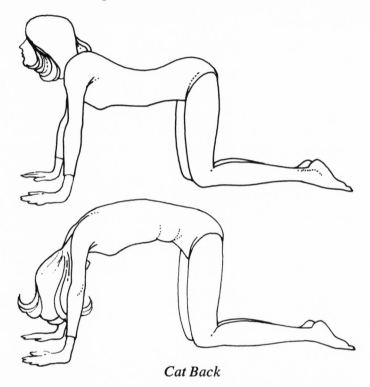

Cat Back

Go down on hands and knees. Tighten stomach muscles, drop head and arch back upward. Then, drop stomach down, and raise head until you are looking straight ahead. Do 4 times. (This increases the flexibility of the spine.)

Stomach Pelvic Tilt

Lie down on stomach, legs close together. Pull stomach off the floor and contract buttocks at the same time. Hold. Relax. Repeat 4 times.

Arm and Leg Raise

Lie on stomach, arms above head. Raise right arm up as high as it can go, keeping it near to ears as you raise it. Do 4 times with each arm, alternating back and forth. Then, lift one leg up slowly; return to starting position. Do 4 times with each leg, alternating back and forth.

Easy Leg Raise

Lie down, arms at sides, legs straight and on floor. Raise right leg up as far as possible; return to starting position. Then, raise left leg; return to starting position. Continue alternating legs and do 4 times with each leg.

12

Exercises to Do in Places You Never Thought of

Exercises don't have to be done only in a special place at a special time. You can work on a wide variety of movements while you're killing time in the most unexpected places: the bathtub, a plane, in bed, waiting in line, while you're hung up on long telephone calls at your desk. Not only will these exercises relieve the bore-dom of the waiting game and make use of those pockets of spare seconds, but they will relieve tension, fight fatigue, and act as mini shape-ups, depending on which you choose to do and where you do them.

At the Beach

Don't just lie there—do something. These exercises can make those long, glorious hours at the beach work for your body, not just your tan.

Foot Flexer

In a standing position, separate toes and stretch upward; then dig toes down into sand. Scrape toes back and forth against sand.

Repeat again and again, alternately stretching and relaxing. This will help to strengthen feet and improve their flexibility.

Sand Builder

Stand up, arms at sides, feet wide apart. Point toes toward each other and slowly push them against the sand, moving feet toward each other as you do so. Next, point heels toward each other and push against sand. Alternate back and forth, pushing toes and heels against sand until feet are almost together. By this time you should have a little pile of sand between your feet. This exercise helps firm inner thighs.

The Lotus Bounce

Sit down with knees bent and pointing outward, soles of feet pressed together and close to your body. Grasp feet with both hands and bounce forward 4 times. Return to starting position and bounce knees up and down 4 times. Repeat sequence 4 times.

Sand Walk

When walking along the beach, slowly push the sand with your toes, alternating from foot to foot. Good for firming thighs and foot flexibility.

Giant Steps

Walk along the sand, taking lunge-type "giant steps," bringing knee up toward chest as you do so. This helps to tone thighs.

On a Plane

Sitting on a plane for even a few hours can make you irritable, tired, cramped up. By doing these exercises every hour or so, you'll rev up your circulation and un-tense your muscles.

Airplane Energizer

In your plane seat, stretch arms overhead and inhale as you do so; then, exhale slowly, simultaneously bringing arms and head down, so that head ends up between knees. Repeat 5 times. This helps fight airplane fatigue by stimulating circulation and encouraging more oxygen intake.

Arm Embrace

In your plane seat, wrap right arm around neck so that it almost touches center of back. Pull elbow to left. (You should feel a stretch when doing this.) Do with left arm. Do with both arms, crossing to do so. Repeat exercise at least 3 times. This stretches your upper back and shoulders and relieves tension.

Feet Treat

A) In plane seat, with feet on floor, stretch toes upward, going back on heels. Return to flat foot position. Then, lift heels by going upward on tiptoe. Repeat 10 times. B) Next, cross legs and circle top ankle slowly 10 times in each direction. Switch cross and repeat with other ankle. These exercises will minimize any swelling caused by sitting for a long period of time because they will pump blood back to the heart.

Jet-Set Stretchers

A) In your plane seat, hold arms out in front of you at shoulder level, parallel to floor, wrists hanging down limply. Stretch fingers up toward ceiling and bring back to touch shoulders. Return to starting position. Repeat at least 5 times. B) Tilt head sideways, so you touch ear to shoulder. Repeat on other side; then, tilt head backward and forward. Repeat 5 times. C) Stand and raise slowly up on toes; relax, and do the Stand-Up Pelvic Tilt (see "Waiting on Line," page 96), so stomach and buttocks get a little action. Do 5 times. This entire series should be done whenever you feel cramped and tired.

At Your Desk

Sure, you can get up and walk around when you want to stretch out, but these chair exercises are designed specifically for those parts of your body that are most affected by desk work. Try one or two whenever you get the chance.

The Shoulder Shrug

Lift left shoulder to ear; bring back to normal position. Repeat with right shoulder. Then, move both shoulders together. Next, do shoulder circles, moving one shoulder at a time in a circular motion, going both backward and forward. Finish up by moving both shoulders together. Great for relieving neck and shoulder tension.

Eye Roll

Picture a clock on the wall in front of you, and with your eyes wide open, focus on each number of the clock, holding each time for a count of 5. Repeat and then do counterclockwise, 2 more times. (If you are doing this correctly, you should be seeing different things as you move around the clock.) This helps relieve eyestrain.

Leg Un-Cramper

Stretch one leg out in front of you and hold for a count of 5. Bring back to starting position. Repeat with other leg. Then do both legs together. Repeat 5 times.

Back Stretcher

Turn to the right, grabbing back of your chair with both arms. Return to center and turn to the left. Repeat 5 times on each side. This exercise helps alleviate back strain.

In the Shower

Make your shower even more reviving by trying these exercises. They're quick and easy and very good for relieving tension.

The Chin Roll

With your back to the shower head, position yourself so that the water hits the back of your neck and shoulders. Pull forward, chin to chest, and hold for a count of 5. Straighten up and rotate chin from right shoulder, down to chest, to left shoulder and back again. Repeat 3 times.

Arm and Shoulder Stretch

In the same position as above exercise, clasp hands behind you. Roll shoulders back and simultaneously bring arms up. Then, lower arms and roll chin forward to chest. Do very slowly. Repeat 3 times, then turn around and repeat again, so that water hits chest. Do entire series very slowly and in a flowing motion.

In the Tub

A long, luxurious soak in the tub is one of the nicest, most relaxing thing you can do for yourself. And it can be a treat for your muscles, as well as your psyche, if you take advantage of the heat's relaxing effect on your muscles, and try the exercises here. They're designed to relieve tension and soothe tired muscles.

The Deep Breather

In a comfortable sitting position, inhale through nose to a count of 5, hold breath for a count of 5, then exhale to a count of 6 through mouth. As you inhale, stomach should expand; as you exhale, stomach should deflate. Concentrate on the counts and the movement of your stomach and repeat again and again. As this series becomes easier, increase your count (inhale 6, exhale

7; inhale 7, exhale 8; and so on) until you reach an inhale count of 15.

Tub Relaxer

Slide back and brace weight on lower arms so that water covers chest. Do Pelvic Tilt (see Basic Pelvic Tilt, Chapter 9—Posture/Balance Fixers). Then, flex feet and rotate ankles. Roll head back and forth. Relax for a count of 5. Repeat. Do at least 3 times.

Body Massage

Sitting with knees slightly bent, slowly knead the muscles of your feet. Separate toes and knead from the base of toes to heel. Then, move up legs, continuing kneading motion and shaking calves with hands to loosen muscles. Continue up to thighs and gently grab and knead them. Next, knead stomach gently. Then, do shoulders, kneading left shoulder with right hand, right shoulder with left. Finish by massaging neck muscles with tips of fingers, rotating upward into hairline. (Note: Do not massage legs if you have varicose veins.)

In Bed

If you have a hard time getting up in the morning, these exercises are made for you. Do them slowly and easily and you'll feel your whole body waking up.

The Joint Stretcher

Lying on back, stretch all the joints of your body, starting with your feet. Point toe, flex ankle of right foot; repeat with left. Tighten and relax each knee. Move each shoulder up and down. Roll head from side to side. Raise arms up toward ceiling and move each wrist backward and forward. Tighten and relax each elbow. Inhale and exhale deeply a few times.

Knee Bounce

Lying on back, with bent knees, feet on bed, rest right foot on left knee and bounce right knee up and down. (You should feel stretch in inner thigh.) Repeat with left leg. Return to starting position. Next, grab right knee with arms and pull it back, pressing it into chest. Repeat with left knee.

Hip Lift

Lying on back with arms at sides and knees bent, lift hips up slowly and return to starting position. Repeat 4 times.

Knee Touch

In same starting position, slowly bring one knee to nose and nose to knee. Return to starting position. Repeat with other leg. Alternate back and forth, 4 times, with each leg.

Waiting on Line

Nothing can be more boring than waiting on line. Why not use those minutes to improve your posture and balance?

Stand-Up Pelvic Tilt

Contract buttocks, tighten abdomen. Release. Repeat again and again, trying to tighten up more forcefully each time. (To make sure you are doing this properly, see the Basic Pelvic Tilt, Chapter 9, Posture/Balance Fixers. Body should be moving in same way.)

Shoulder-to-Shoulder

Standing tall, pull shoulder blades together, then slump forward. Repeat 5 times.

Knee Flexer

Just tighten and release knees again and again. This helps strengthen thighs.

Balance Improver

Lift one foot just an inch above ground. Tighten stomach muscles, but don't hold breath, and keep foot raised for a count of 5. Return foot to ground and repeat on other leg. Do as often as you like.

13

Situation Chart

The following chart will give you an idea of how to plan and change around your program to suit your specific needs. It lists eight typical working woman's problems and a specially designed routine to fit each. Look it over to get an understanding of how to plan your own program and flip back to it whenever you're caught in one of the problem situations. Keep in mind, however, that this is a guideline and you are free to substitute other exercises from this book if you have found they better meet your individual needs in a particular situation.

(Note: The reason a few of these routines don't add up to the 13-minute recommendation is that they're only once-in-a-while situations, not regular workouts. Your basic routine, however, should total at least 90 minutes weekly.)

Situation	Time	Program	Reason
MAD AS HELL	14–16 min.	1 min. Basic Body Relaxer (Ch. 4) 2 min. Tension Releasers (Ch. 8) 2 min. Jogger (Ch. 4) 3–5 min. Bouncing Body Chorus Line Kick } (Ch. 6) Knee Bend & Kick 3 min. Figure Improvers of your choice (Ch. 5) 1 min. Pectoral Stretch } (Ch. 7) Rocking Horse 2 min. Rag Doll series (Ch. 10)	Because these exercises require a good amount of movement and much exertion, they will help release tension.
HARD DAY AHEAD	10–11 min.	2 min. "In Bed" Exercises (Ch. 12) 1 min. Warm-Ups for People Who Are on Their Feet All Day (Ch. 4) 4½ min. Basic Sit-Up Lift & Stretch Knee Bounce Inner Thigh Pull } (Ch. 5) Waist Circles Body Twister The Arc Arm Circles	This workout, which starts off with lying down exercises, will get your blood circulating and wake you up in an easy, non-strenuous way.

Situation	Time	Program	Reason
HARD DAY AHEAD (cont'd)		Calf Exercises (Ch. 5)	
		½ min. Ankle Flexer ⎫ Zipper Pull ⎬ (Ch. 7) ⎭	
		2 min. Rag Doll series (Ch. 10)	
OFFICE-TO-DATE	10 minutes (not including shower)	1 min. Basic Body Relaxer (Ch. 4)	This "refresher workout" takes only a short time and is a great way to unwind and get your second wind.
		2 min. Tension Releasers (Ch. 8)	
		2 min. Warm-Ups—choose which series applies to you (Ch. 4)	
		4 min. Sit-Up Twist Leg Forward Stretch Knee Bounce ⎫ Tippy-Toe Raise ⎬ (Ch. 5) Studio Twist Waist Circles ⎭	
		½ min. Shoulder Pull (Ch. 7)	
		½ min. Crab Walk (Ch. 6)	
		End with a quick shower, where you do the "In the Shower" exercises (Ch. 12)	
KINKED UP AND STIFF	14 minutes	1 min. Basic Body Relaxer (Ch. 4)	This is basically a "stretching" routine and will move joints in all
		2 min. Warm-Ups for People Who Are on Their Feet All Day (Ch. 4)	

directions and extend muscles to their full length. Result: stiffness is eased, muscles relaxed.

½ min. Shoulder Pull (Ch. 7)
½ min. Cat-Back (Ch. 11)
5 min. Flexibility Exercises of your choice, but include Back Stretcher (Ch. 7)

1 min. Back Strengtheners (Ch. 9)
2 min. Menstrual Soothers (Ch. 11)
2 min. Rag Doll series (Ch. 10)

HARD DAY AT THE OFFICE — 13 minutes

This routine releases tension and loosens up stiff muscles, as well as working on "office spread."

5 min. Tension Releasers (Ch. 8)
2 min. Jazzaerobics (Ch. 4)
3 min. Basic Sit-Up } (Ch. 5)
      Triple Threat }
½ min. Balance Improvers (Ch. 9)
½ min. Rest Position (Ch. 4)
2 min. Sit Down Coolers (Ch. 10)

ON YOUR FEET ALL DAY — 12–13 minutes

Since most of this program is done lying down with feet up, it will re-

2 min. Basic Body Relaxer (Ch. 4)
2 min. Warm-Ups for People Who Are on Their Feet All Day (Ch. 4)

Situation	Time	Program	Reason
ON YOUR FEET ALL DAY (cont'd)		½ min. Basic Sit-Up ½ min. Diagonal Leg Lift 1 min. Lift & Switch 1 min. The Crossover } (Ch. 5) 1 min. Hip Roll 1 min. Arm & Bust Exercises, including Basic Push-Up 1 min. Heel Stretcher 　　　Foot Clapper } (Ch. 7) 　　　Foot Thrust 　　　Bend & Twist } 2 min. Lazy Woman's Cool-Offs (Ch. 10)	lieve pressure on feet and start circulation going upward toward head.
"I'VE NEVER EXERCISED BEFORE"	15–17 minutes	5 min. Tension Releasers (Ch. 8) ½ min. Basic Pelvic Tilt (Ch. 9) 2 min. Warm-Ups for People Who Are on Their Feet All Day (Ch. 4)— end with Rest Position 5 min. Basic Sit-Up 　　　(do with arms over head) } (Ch. 5) 　　　Lift & Switch 　　　The Crossover }	This is a "beginner" program which will stretch muscles gradually and ease you gently into a familiarity with exercises. Once you've mastered it, build from there and create your own program.

Triple Threat
Basic Push-Up
Any Arm & Bust Exercises } (Ch. 5)
Calf Exercises

½ min. Heel Stretch } (Ch. 7)
Back Stretcher

2 min. Lazy Woman's Cool-Offs (Ch. 10)

ON THE ROAD
(or, how to exercise
in a hotel room while
attending a convention,
sales conference, etc.)

13 min.

5 min. Tension Release program (Ch. 8)

2 min. Jazzaerobic Warm-Ups (Ch. 4)

½ min. Bouncing Body—finish with Rest Position (Ch. 6)

2 min. Basic Sit-Up
Leg Extension } (Ch. 5)
Single Leg Lift

1½ min. Heel Stretch
Sole Clapper } (Ch. 7)
Back Stretcher

2 min. Rag Doll series (Ch. 10)

This is a great unkinker routine. It starts off by relaxing your muscles, then gets your blood circulating and stretches your ligaments. It can also be done in a small space.

14

The Working Woman's Diet

All the exercise in the world isn't going to do much good if you don't eat correctly. But just what *is* good eating? Most doctors agree that the best diet—whether you want to lose, gain, or maintain weight—is a low-carbohydrate, high-protein one. Such a diet includes lots of fish and chicken, some lean meat, plus fresh fruits and vegetables with limited sugars and fats. And, yes, calories *do* count. If you eat more calories than you use up for heat and energy, you gain weight; if you use up more than you eat, you lose. In order to get rid of one pound of fat, you must cut out (or work off with activity) 3500 calories. To figure out how many calories you should consume to lose weight, multiply your present weight by 15. That's the amount of calories needed daily to maintain your weight. Cut back by 500 a day and you'll lose a pound a week.

Sounds easy, but as anyone who's ever tried to diet knows, it isn't. And when you're a working woman—with a working woman's busy, ever changing, often frustrating, lifestyle—it's almost impossible. One night at class someone casually remarked to another student, a home ec teacher, "Hey, Kaye, you're getting a tummy." She burst into tears and said she was gaining weight because "There's food wherever I look." Well, my class immediately turned into a sympathetic rap session about the obstacles working sets up to eating healthfully. For instance, how do you cope with business meals? So much of business today is conducted around eating or drinking that you cannot stick to a typical day-by-day menu diet. Then, there are those hectic days when you can't even get out to sit down and order a low-calorie lunch and have to grab something on the run or from the coffee wagon instead. And what do you cook when you get home late and the kids are screaming for dinner—"now"?

It is discouraging, but there is an answer. By changing your eating habits just a bit, planning ahead, and avoiding the really fat-rich foods, you can lose and still live well. This chapter will show you how—and not with a strict diet plan, but with tips chosen to fit the working woman's lifestyle and special problems.

How to Diet Successfully

The first rule of dieting for a working woman is not to take off too much too fast. Do that and you lose energy, which is bound to show up in your job performance. Go slowly and don't expect miracles. Studies have shown that the most successful dieters lose two pounds a week, tops. It doesn't sound like much, but the weight loss is steady and tends to be permanent.

The second rule is to be prepared for fluctuations and plateaus in weight. Retention of water in the body, food in the stomach, the amount of water lost through perspiration and daily kidney and intestinal functions can make your body weight vary a few pounds. Furthermore, your pattern of weight loss might not be steady. Sometimes your tissues and skin may not shrink back as fast as the fat is being lost and the resulting "empty space" gets filled with water. Eventually, the underlying tissues and skin will shrink and the fluid will stop accumulating. Then, too, weight is affected by activity and, in periods when you are less active, you'll probably experience a temporary slowing of weight loss.

Another important guideline of successful dieting is to eat slowly and chew food well. If this sounds like your mother talking, well, mom is right. When you gulp food down, you won't feel satisfied because *it takes at least 20 minutes for the stomach to signal the brain that it is satisfied.* Eating fast also tempts you to have seconds. One student, who fights a daily battle with gaining weight, has found that eating with chopsticks forces her to eat more slowly. I always put my spoon or fork down between mouthfuls so I won't gobble. And, when eating out, I always tell the waiter to serve the courses slowly—besides being a more pleasant way to eat, I find that I don't eat as much. Edith, a magazine editor who was gaining weight because people were constantly taking her to lunch, tried this and loves it because "it doesn't give me any time to eat dessert." Following are some more guidelines that you can easily apply to your working lifestyle:

· Maintain a fairly constant calorie intake rather than the yo-yo kind of dieting where you alternately starve and gorge. The latter is not only unhealthy, it rarely results in a permanent weight loss.

· Many women eat too many calories because they are not aware of calorie traps. Buy a good pocket calorie counter and read it. Look up your favorite foods and see if you can find lower-calorie substitutes.

· Start a diet when you're "up." If things are going wrong, you've just changed jobs, or you're up for a promotion, it will be harder to watch your calories because you'll be worrying about other things.

· Be assertive. Eat only what *you* want and don't let other people sabotage your diet. You must learn to say "no." I have, and believe me, I haven't lost any friends in the process. Many women use the "Well, he/she insisted" line as an excuse to indulge their own desires.

· Try eating four or five mini-meals a day, rather than limiting yourself to three. Because you'll be eating more often, you won't have as much of a desire to nibble.

· Listen to your stomach and eat only when hungry. Remember that hunger is different from appetite. Hunger is your body's signal for food and it usually registers as pangs in your stomach; appetite is a highly emotional state that's based on the pleasure of eating. You're intelligent enough to know when your mind is signaling you and not your body.

· Be sure to include fiber in your diet. It is needed to make the digestive system function at its peak. Without it, you won't have proper elimination. High fiber foods are unprocessed fruits and vegetables, wheat germ, bran flakes, whole grain bread, soy beans, lentils.

· Don't skip breakfast. Even though your body has been in a fasting state while sleeping, it's still been burning up calories for heat and your energy reserves need to be replenished to put you in peak shape for your working day. This doesn't mean you need to eat a huge country breakfast, but have something to get you going. A cut-up orange sprinkled with coconut, granola with honey, plain yogurt with berries, a piece of cheese with fresh fruit and a couple of crackers—all of these are easy to fix, tempting, and nutritious.

· Get enough sleep. Willpower weakens with fatigue.

· If you're a snacker, save part of your lunch to satisfy your growling stomach at 3 o'clock or your dessert from dinner for a before-bed snack.

· Trim excess fat off meat and use lean ground round or lean sirloin in place of the fatter ground meats for hamburgers.

· Have a cup of bouillon when you come home from work to put those "6 o'clock hunger pangs" to rest; then eat dinner later.

The Cottage Cheese Crash

One of the hardest parts of dieting is to get started. This mini-diet is easy to handle because it doesn't involve much preparation (good if you're single and eating alone or married and need to prepare another meal for your family) and the loss it will register on your scale is the best encouragement there is to keep counting calories. What's more, you're only on it for a day or two, so you can stick to it without much of a hassle. Follow it on days when you don't have business or social dates. It's for you to eat at your desk and at home when you're not entertaining.

Breakfast: One 8-oz. container of cottage cheese, one slice of diet bread or two rye crisps; coffee or tea with no sugar

Lunch: One 8-oz. container of cottage cheese with an 8-oz. can of diet fruit (apricots, pears, peaches); coffee or tea with no sugar

Dinner: One 8-oz. container of cottage cheese with lettuce, cucumber, or endive. Also, up to 2 cups of one of the following vegetables, either raw or cooked: as-

paragus, spinach, stringbeans, or broccoli. Use 1
tbsp. diet dressing on the salad. Dessert: an apple or
pear; coffee or tea with no sugar

Drink at least 4 glasses of water during the day.

If you don't finish up all three containers of cottage cheese, have
what's left over as a snack before going to bed. Also, have a
grapefruit any time during the day to stave off hunger pangs,
and a carrot or piece of celery before dinner.

If you're going out of your mind on the second day, have a glass
of wine with dinner.

The rest of the week eat a normal diet, sensibly limiting your
carbohydrates and fats.

Repeat the two-day diet for two more weeks if you still want to
lose weight.

The Working Woman's Diet Traps—and How to Beat Them

The Business Meal

This is a definite calorie trap. You usually feel obligated to
keep up with the other person, and because the money isn't out
of your pocket, might be tempted to fill up on dishes you otherwise wouldn't order. Keep these suggestions in mind the next
time a business lunch comes up.

· Order a clear soup or tomato juice as an appetizer. Either of
these will give you something to concentrate on while others
are eating more fattening dishes. They'll also help to keep you
away from the bread and butter.
· Avoid ordering casseroles or other mixed dishes. They almost
always contain a lot of fattening carbohydrates, creamed soups,
or sauces.
· For your main dish, have broiled poultry, grilled fish "dry," or
a salad with a freshly squeezed lemon for dressing.
· Have either a potato or a roll, not both.
· Speak up. Ask the waiter to bring the meat without the gravy
or sauce, ask for salad dressing on the side, ask for unbuttered
vegetables.
· Stay away from fried foods, cream sauces, creamed soups.
· Remember you don't have to eat everything on your plate.

- Limit yourself to a glass of wine or one drink. Or, better yet, order Perrier water with a slice of lime.
- If you get to choose the restaurant, pick a Chinese or seafood establishment rather than Italian or French. Another good choice is a restaurant that specializes in steak or "grills" because you won't have to worry about rich sauces.
- Order espresso coffee instead of dessert.
- If you must succumb to a dessert, eat only half. After all, the second half tastes the same and only ends up doubling the calories.

Brown-Bagging It

Everyone brown bags it at some time or other, but you'd probably do it more often if you could think of some interesting eats to put in the bag. Here are some good ones:

- Pack a frozen shrimp or crabmeat cocktail in the morning and by lunch it will be thawed, but still cool. Eat with saltines, rye crackers, or melba toast. Finish up with a piece of fresh fruit.
- Plain cottage cheese is a bore, but add chunks of fresh pineapple and raisins, chopped scallions, chives and green olives, or a few chopped up radishes, walnuts, and black olives, and you've got an appetizing dish.
- If you're a sandwich freak, use 2 slices of diet- or thin-sliced bread to save about 30 calories.
- For a delicious brown-bag salad, do this the night before: Place lettuce or spinach leaves on a foil pie plate and top with slices of chopped egg, mushrooms and cucumbers, shredded carrot, a cubed tomato, a few artichoke hearts, some crunchy bean sprouts. Wrap in foil, refrigerate overnight, and bag in the morning along with either a fresh lemon (to squeeze for dressing) or an aspirin bottle filled with diet dressing. You can also do a similar thing with fresh fruit—just cut up the fruit the night before, coat anything that might turn with lemon juice, and use vanilla yogurt as dressing.
- Try the un-sandwich: Wrap cold slices of chicken, roast beef, or turkey in foil; put a tomato, hunk of cheese, and some sliced raw mushrooms into a plastic bag; add a pear for dessert.
- By all means bag your yogurt, but make it the plain variety. Freeze in its carton overnight. When lunchtime comes around,

add your own fruit, berries, or instant coffee or vanilla extract for flavoring. It's cheaper and more fun than buying ready-made flavored yogurt.

· A tomato stuffed with egg, tuna, or chicken salad is a good brown bag idea, but make the salad with yogurt instead of mayo—it saves calories.

· Keep the following little extras in your desk to make your brown bag eats more tempting: salt and a pepper mill, small jar of grated parmesan, small bottle of lemon juice, packages of melba toast, a few boxes of raisins, some pill bottles filled with freeze-dried chives, oregano, paprika, and curry powder, and bags of dried fruits.

· Two good investments if you brown bag it often are an immersion heater and a thermos. Use the heater to cook up packaged dried or one-serving canned soup, as well as coffee and tea; pack the thermos with luscious cold soups like gazpacho or avocado soup, or whip up your favorite health drink in the morning and put that in the thermos.

Eating on the Run

You probably run into this problem at least a few times a month; you're very busy, have no time to grab a bite, but you're famished and need the energy. What to do? Look over these suggestions:

· Buy one of the diet snack packs available at most candy stores. They're made of a mixture of nuts and dried fruits and are a good, quick way to tide you over the next few hours.

· Pass up the fast-food burger and fried chicken chains, and have a slice of pizza instead. It's a good source of protein, B vitamins, and vitamin F, and comes in at around 200 calories. If you do stop at a burger chain, choose the cheapest burger. It's not only the lowest in price, but in fat and calories. Even better are the fish sandwiches—just tell them to skip the special sauce and garnishes.

· Stop at the deli and buy a piece of cheese. Nibble on it and a box of raisins or an apple or some dried fruit.

· Do not buy a candy bar. It will give you fast energy, yes, but the energy lift will only last a short time. What really happens is that the sugar in the candy will cause your blood sugar to rise (instant energy) for a couple of hours, but then it will drop and you will feel even more fatigued.

· If you have time, stop at a coffee shop and order soup and a salad. Or have a sandwich, but eat only one slice of bread and use mustard instead of mayo.

· If you know you have an action-packed day ahead, do not, repeat, do not skip breakfast. You need it as a source of energy.

· Any of the many snack or breakfast bars is a good, nutritious way to eat on the run. Supplement with an apple or pear and you'll be good for hours.

Dinner for One

Eating dinner alone can be a hazard because you're apt to snack on chips or cookies instead of making a nutritious meal. Or, you'll opt for something that heats up quickly, like noodles or a casserole, and regret the calories later. Here are some ideas for nutritious, non-fattening, one-woman meals.

· Make yourself a promise to eat a real meal, one that contains some protein and some carbohydrates. This doesn't necessarily mean something elaborate—broil a steak or piece of fish and eat with a salad, toss a huge salad and supplement it with soup, make a low-calorie vegetable dish ahead of time and serve as a side dish with a piece of chicken.

· Stop on the way home from work, pick up some beautiful greens and make a fabulous salad. Two suggestions: a spinach salad made with raw spinach leaves, sliced raw mushrooms, imitation bacon bits and a hard-boiled egg and diet dressing; or a Chinese salad made with Chinese cabbage leaves and mustard greens, bean sprouts, scallions, raw mushrooms, water chestnuts, and sesame seeds, served with a mustard soy-sauce dressing. With your salad have a glass of wine and a scoop of sherbet or ice milk for dessert.

· Stock up on some nutritious convenience foods so you aren't tempted to nibble on potato chips. Include fillings for omelettes (mushrooms, cheese, artichoke hearts, stewed tomatoes, and zucchini), canned goods like tuna, crabmeat, soup, water-packed fruits; frozen vegetables, shrimp, fish fillets; diet breakfast or snack bars; vegetable and fruit juices; raisins, bouillon cubes, vitamin-fortified cereals.

- Learn how to use herbs and spices. They're a good way to add flavor, but not calories, to almost anything.
- Practice making the perfect omelette. Once you've mastered the technique, you can fill your omelettes with all sorts of things and have a very good meal. Some good fillers are: asparagus and Cheddar cheese, cottage cheese and chives, sautéed vegetables such as tomatoes, onions, and zucchini, refried beans, Swiss cheese and raisins, mozzarella, dietetic jelly.
- Plan activities while you're waiting for dinner to cook—standing around in the kitchen only tempts you to raid the refrigerator. Polish your toenails, iron clothes for the next day, balance your checkbook.
- Any of these quick-cook ideas are well worth trying: sprinkle a piece of fish with tarragon and fresh pepper, squeeze a lemon over it, pop into the broiler and serve with slices of lemon; cover a chicken breast with a mixture of curry powder, crushed garlic, onion salt, fresh pepper and broil it, adding green pepper rings and scallions or shallots when halfway through; sauté bean sprouts with a crushed garlic cube, sliced mushrooms and diced scallions and soy sauce (good with steak or chicken); sauté shrimp until pink and serve with sautéed slivered almonds and chives.

Eating with Your Family

When you have children and/or a husband to worry about, you don't have as much leeway with the foods you prepare. You might be satisfied with a salad, but they're apt to sniff at that and demand meat and potatoes. Here are some ways to cut calories, and still keep the family happy:

- Sauté foods with chicken broth, soy sauce, or wine, instead of oil or butter. Lemon juice is another good substitute.
- Use dietetic jams, jellies, syrups, and sodas. No one will know the difference.
- Eat the same dishes as everyone else, but make smaller portions for yourself. Pass up breads, sugars, and starches.
- Broil or bake your meats; fry in no-stick pans or use one of the spray-on coatings that have fewer calories than butter.
- Cut back on fatty, high-calorie meats like pork, lamb, most beef. Add more fish and poultry to your meals.

· Eat a salad before your meal to fill you up before you get to the high-calorie stuff. For dressing, just use salt and pepper, a squeeze of lemon juice, and a sprinkle of Parmesan cheese.
· Make it a habit to use butter salt instead of butter, plain yogurt instead of sour cream.
· Bone up on East Indian and Turkish cuisine. Both use lots of yogurt and fresh vegetables and are less fattening than most Italian and French dishes.
· Instead of serving cake or pastry for dessert, try fresh berries, fruit, sherbet, ice milk.
· Buy a low-calorie cookbook, use the recipes, and don't tell anyone. Your husband and children probably won't notice anything different.
· Make smart substitutions to save calories: try poached eggs instead of scrambled, puffed rice for rice flakes, club steak for meat loaf, pretzels for potato chips, grapes for peanuts, beef bouillon for creamed soup.
· Cut out the cakes and cookies. They're bad for you and your family and your desire for them is probably based on habit more than anything else. If you start now, you'll be doing a favor for your children because they won't get used to having them around.

The Party/Liquor Predicament

Sales conferences, business lunches, conventions, receptions, even "let's talk about this over a drink" can be a dieter's downfall. Left to roam among the trays of hors d'oeuvres or sitting next to a bowl of peanuts, you're bound to slip up. These tips will help.

· When ordering a drink, keep in mind that wine is much lower in calories than hard liquor. And mixed drinks total in at much more than those with water or on-the-rocks.
· Diluting liquor with water slows down the absorption rate; mixing it with a carbonated beverage speeds up the absorption rate.
· If you don't want to drink, or want something very light, try Perrier, a white wine spritzer, Campari with a twist.
· At a party, scout around before you start to nibble. Once you know what is available, choose the least caloric and ration yourself.

· Shrimp, crudités, olives, and cheeses are the best hors d'oeuvres bets. Don't even look at the chips and dips, the sugary nuts, the elegant concoctions made with cream cheese, sour cream, or mayonnaise.

· Don't skip meals the day of the party. Going without lunch or dinner won't save calories at all because you'll end up being so starved that you'll gorge on all the fattening hors d'oeuvres. Better to eat lightly—say soup and salad for dinner if it's a late party, or grilled fish and a vegetable for lunch if it's an early bash.

· If you have absolutely no will power, try this trick: Stick a bag of dried fruits in your pocketbook and when your stomach starts to growl, munch on them in the bathroom. They'll fill up that hole in your stomach and help you to resist temptation.

Exercise and Weight Loss

Besides counting your calories and limiting your fat and carbohydrate intake, try to get as much exercise as possible. For every minute of physical activity you take part in, your body burns up calories and the more exercise you get (and the more effort you put into it), the faster you'll lose weight. It's also true that activity relieves boredom and since boredom often leads to overeating, you'll have less time and reason to think about food. In fact, many experiments have indicated that most people experience a definite loss of appetite once they start exercising regularly.

The following chart lists some common activities and shows how far they go in burning up calories. Keep it in mind the next time you eat a Big Mac and are tempted to take the bus home instead of walking.

(Note: Quantities given are approximate. Much depends on the individual's weight and metabolism, the effort expended, the speed.)

activity	calories burned (per hour)	food equivalent
exercises in this book	500	1 chocolate malted (8 oz.)
sitting, typing	90	6 cocktail shrimp with sauce
strolling (1 mph)	120	1 cup chicken noodle soup
walking (2 mph)	200	1 piece of fudge
tennis (singles)	450	1 piece chocolate cake with icing
dancing (fast)	350	hamburger on a bun
skiing (moderate pace)	600	1 Burger King Whopper
swimming (moderate pace)	450	1 piece coconut cream pie
jogging (5 mph)	500	1 turkey sandwich with gravy
cycling (13 mph)	650	3 pieces Kentucky Fried chicken
bowling	250	1 ice cream soda
ironing	100	2 slices bacon
vacuuming, mopping	285	hot dog on a bun with sauerkraut
scrubbing floors	360	1 average serving flank steak
watching TV	80	1 glass skim milk (8 oz.)

Epilogue

Well, that about sums it up. You have my program—now it's up to you. Remember, if by some chance you start to get bored, change the exercises—fast.

Expect to see definite results in 6 to 8 weeks, but realize that some areas respond more quickly than others. One thing is certain, though—if you work out regularly, you'll soon feel better all over. Exercise increases your sense of well-being, helps fight fatigue, reduces susceptibility to disease, and builds up your energy reserves. Add all that to a better-toned and better-looking body, and you've got a lot of reasons to keep at it!

As a parting comment, I want to repeat something that one of my clients who has been coming to my studio for ten years said when she heard about this book. "I'm so glad. Exercising with you has done me a world of good. I've just turned forty and look better now than I did at thirty. Maybe with this book, other women can look forward to that, too."

I certainly hope so.

Index

119